WALK THIS WAY

THE PROVEN "STEP-BY-STEP" LOW IMPACT EXERCISE GUIDE TO LOSE WEIGHT, EASE ANXIETY, INCREASE PRODUCTIVITY, AND REGAIN YOUR HEALTH

PARKER SCRIPPS, M.A.

© **Copyright 2023 - All rights reserved.**

The content contained within this book may not be reproduced, duplicated or transmitted without direct written permission from the author or the publisher.

Under no circumstances will any blame or legal responsibility be held against the publisher, or author, for any damages, reparation, or monetary loss due to the information contained within this book, either directly or indirectly.

Legal Notice:

This book is copyright protected. It is only for personal use. You cannot amend, distribute, sell, use, quote or paraphrase any part, or the content within this book, without the consent of the author or publisher.

Disclaimer Notice:

Please note the information contained within this document is for educational and entertainment purposes only. All effort has been executed to present accurate, up to date, reliable, complete information. No warranties of any kind are declared or implied. Readers acknowledge that the author is not engaged in the rendering of legal, financial, medical or professional advice. The content within this book has been derived from various sources. Please consult a licensed professional before attempting any techniques outlined in this book.

By reading this document, the reader agrees that under no circumstances is the author responsible for any losses, direct or indirect, that are incurred as a result of the use of the information contained within this document, including, but not limited to, errors, omissions, or inaccuracies.

CONTENTS

Introduction   5

1. A WALKTHROUGH OF EXERCISE WALKING   15
   Walking Improves Your Physical Health   17
   Walking Improves Your Mental Health   27
   Determining Your Baseline Condition   33

2. WALK AWAY YOUR WORRIES   43
   Other Surprising Benefits of Walking   52

3. FIRST STEPS   63
   Shoe Shopping   65
   Walking Safety   77
   Warming Up and Cooling Down   81

4. WALKING TECHNIQUE AND SETTING YOUR OWN PACE   99
   Benefits of Proper Posture and Good Walking Technique   100
   Creating Sustainability   113

5. ENJOYING THE GREAT OUTDOORS   121
   Why Walk Outdoors?   123
   Outdoor Walking Exercises   126

6. WALKING INDOORS   133
   Indoor Walking Exercises   137

7. GOING A STEP FURTHER   151
   Taking Your Walking Workout to the Next Level   152

8. CREATING YOUR WALKING HABIT   159
   How Do I Create Habits?   161

Conclusion 171
References 175

INTRODUCTION

> *When you have worn out your shoes, the strength of the shoe leather has passed into the fiber of your body. I measure your health by the number of shoes and hats and clothes you have worn out.*
>
> — RALPH WALDO EMERSON

As someone with a background in long-distance running, competitive sports, and tennis during my high school and college years, I never thought that I would fall off the fitness wagon. The image of myself as a strong, healthy, vibrant individual remained in my mind for several decades, through family and career transitions and beyond. This all changed, of course, when I reached my mid-40s and began feeling winded climbing a single flight of stairs. When I routinely felt sore and weak after half-mile walks, the vision of myself as a young, healthy 20-year-old came crashing down around me. My self-esteem plummeted, and my career and motivation suddenly seemed to hit a wall. I asked myself how, after years of training, could I have come to this point?

After consulting with friends and family around my age, I quickly came to the realization that it wasn't just me—nearly everyone I knew nearing middle age felt tired, worn down, and weaker than ever. Rationally, of course, I knew that I would lose energy as I got older; but experiencing such an unexpected sensation of unwelcome aging was worse than I had imagined. Not only was I out of shape, but I also felt a stunning lack of motivation to do anything about it.

It was here I discovered that I had dropped the ball, so to speak—I hadn't been looking. Keeping active when I was young and spry had never been an issue and took very little effort, but I had entirely overlooked the matter of *staying* active as I grew older. Now, middle-aged and in a state of relatively poor physical and mental health, I found that I had lost many of the tools that had made fitness easy for me in the past. I didn't have any workout equipment, I didn't have a gym membership, and I was at a loss about where to start. At this point, trying to play a sport or exercise at a facility was utterly daunting; and even running would have been a big stretch for me. So, with the knowledge that I needed to change my habits soon or risk my health even further, I did the one thing that I knew I could do —I walked. At first, I only walked a couple times per day, in segments of five to seven minutes. During these first outings, I returned home feeling out of breath and heavy from taking just a lap around my block. But, it was a start! Over a period of several weeks, those five minutes became increasingly easier, and I began recording them in a small notebook that I kept on my desk at home.

Five minutes soon grew to ten, which grew to twenty, which then grew to forty-five. In a period of two months, I went from a state of absolute inactivity to being able to walk for an entire hour without feeling exhausted. As it turned out, I didn't need a gym membership or fancy equipment to improve my physical fitness—I only needed to take that first step.

WHY WALKING?

If you're anything like me, the mere prospect of a new health regimen can seem overwhelming. Considering all of the trends and expert opinions we are exposed to through channels like television, print, social media and other platforms, it's no wonder that the prospect of "getting in shape" is so confusing and daunting. To put things in perspective, let's take a look at the health and fitness industry. According to data from Adjust Analytics, a whopping 71,000 new health and fitness apps were launched on Apple and Android app stores in 2020 alone (Wetzler, 2021). And this does not include health and fitness giants like Fitbit, Peloton, and Strava, all of which have been on the market for years. According to one Business of Apps survey, in 2021 the health and fitness app industry generated $5.35 billion from its user base of nearly 400 million customers (Curry, 2023). In fact, if you have Apple or Android products, chances are that you already have some health and fitness resources like pedometers and calorie trackers built into your phone, tablet, or smartwatch. In short, there is a wealth of fitness resources available including the more traditional options of gyms, nutritionists, and personal trainers.

The number of offerings can be baffling. Which to choose? How did the simple act of exercise become so complicated? Humans have been on this planet for thousands of years, staying physically active and eating well. Why is all of this new technology emerging right now? Are apps and smart technology *really* necessary to stay healthy?

The ancient Greeks probably wouldn't think so, nor would ancient Chinese or Indian civilizations. While one's physical health has always been important, the history of fitness has not (until the last 200 years or so) included advanced technology of any kind. In the regions of China and India, activities like gymnastics, dancing, wrestling, and yoga were popular fitness measures—many of which were incorporated into daily life. According to Dr. Len Kravitz of the University of New Mexico, ancient Chinese society during the Confucius era, "recognized that physical inactivity was associated with certain diseases," and these diseases, "were preventable with regular exercise for fitness" (Dalleck & Kravitz, 2019). As a result, a new style of gymnastics was developed to keep the general population healthy. This new style, called Cong Fu, was designed to imitate the movements of different animals in nature, each with its own unique series of motions and positions. During roughly the same period, India and the broader South Asian region were cultivating another form of physical engagement: Yoga.

Approximately 5,000 years ago, the North Indian Indus-Sarasvati Civilization began developing a system of intentional movements to accompany Vedic religious chants. The Vedic texts that detail early forms of yoga (called the Rigveda) are considered some of the most holy texts in Hinduism, which is perhaps why yoga is such a widespread practice in today's world. In addition to religious fulfillment, the practice of yoga was also crafted to keep practitioners physically healthy, with an emphasis on flexibility and strength-building (Ayeh-Datey, 2022).

Pre-Christian fitness practices, however, weren't limited to China and India by any means. Many ancient cultures from around the world crafted their own methods of staying healthy, from the Spartans to the Native Americans. Of course, a skeptic might point to the fact that historic populations were physically fit out of sheer necessity, or for the purposes of war. While we're not hunting and gathering food anymore, I still think Confucius had a good point when he said that, "roads were made for journeys, not destinations" (GoodReads, n.d.-a). Keeping with that metaphor, the destination has certainly changed, but the road has not!

In examining sports and physical activities throughout history, you might have picked up on one glaring commonality—many of these activities require absolutely no equipment. You can dance anywhere you'd like, you can practice martial arts with nothing but your body, and even traditional yoga was actually practiced on the bare ground (Cler, 2015)! That's not to say that you shouldn't invest in good equipment, but fancy machines and complex apps aren't necessary to get in shape. Additionally, many of these ancient activities were created for use by the masses. Cong Fu, for instance, wasn't reserved for the elite or the warrior class. Yoga was, in part, a religious tool to enlighten followers of Hinduism. Everyday people of all classes and ages could take part in fitness measures, and were even actively encouraged to participate.

Luckily, you don't have to be a Cong Fu master or an expert yogi to stay in shape (although both options are a great addition to your repertoire), nor do you need special equipment or a high social status. Despite the fitness trends that circulate every few years, and the countless apps and products that promise instantaneous results, there is only one thing you need in order to keep yourself healthy—You! Wherever you are in your fitness journey, there is probably at least one activity that you can do every day. For many, the most accessible form of physical exercise is also the simplest: walking. While not a high-intensity activity at first glance, walking is a great entry point for those who have preexisting conditions, limiting physical injuries, or other health concerns. Young or old, walking for just a couple of minutes per day is, contrary to popular belief, still a valid form of exercise!

In today's world, it can be tiring to see celebrities on social media constantly touting products and regimens for physical health that will "fix it all". Fortunately, for those of us feeling flooded with advertisements and false promises, there is a wealth of health and wellness knowledge that we can draw upon. No matter what your end goal is, walking is perhaps the easiest and most accessible point of entry into the world of fitness. From weight loss to physical upkeep as you get older, walking is the best basis upon which to build your wellness routine.

No matter what your current capabilities are, the simple activity of walking will provide you with a means of improving yourself. No, you don't have to be dripping with sweat at the end of every workout in order to see results in your quality of life. Take it from Lee Haney, one of the most decorated bodybuilders in American history: "Exercise to stimulate, not to annihilate. The world wasn't formed in a day, and neither were we. Set small goals and build upon them" (BrainyQuote, n.d.). As the saying goes, slow and steady wins the race. The same can be said of your wellness and fitness journey!

In the following chapters, we'll walk through each facet of setting up a sustainable walking routine, step by step. From finding the right shoes to forming a walking community, and everything in between—you'll see that your physical endurance, mental health, and social relationships are bound to prosper. There's only one more question you need to ask yourself: Are you ready to take the first step?

1

A WALKTHROUGH OF EXERCISE WALKING

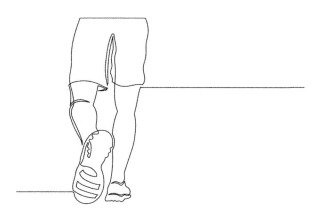

" *Walking gets the feet moving, the blood moving, the mind moving.*

— TERRI GUILLEMETS

On occasion, I'll see fitness content on my Instagram feed. In my case, most of this content revolves around difficult or novel yoga poses that someone has accomplished. Sometimes I'll take out my dust-covered yoga mat to try these maneuvers, only to realize that they are much harder in real life than I thought they'd be. It's usually at this point that I roll up my yoga mat and put it back into its dark corner in my closet, not to be used for the rest of the month.

For me, it's easy to conceptualize fitness, but sometimes very difficult to actually bring myself to stay fit. When an activity requires advanced moves, expensive equipment, or a lot of knowledge of how to do the activity correctly, it can prove to be a massive barrier between you and your health goals. As we touched on in the last chapter, many historical fitness practices prioritized accessibility, which is perhaps why they were (and still are) so popular among the general public. Physical and financial barriers, in addition to making it more difficult to get started, can also potentially discourage you from continuing to be active in the long term. This is the difference between sustainable activity and more temporary health trends and fads that you might see on social media or television.

For most of us, activities such as tennis or pickleball (both involving many rules and equipment prerequisites) is probably not my best option for sustainable fitness. Meanwhile, walking—an activity that many of us do every day anyway—has the potential to carry the same benefits as sports or martial arts. According to the Mayo Clinic, consistently walking at a brisk pace can help you lose fat, manage cardiovascular conditions, and even strengthen your immune system (Mayo Clinic Staff, 2021b). Unfortunately, much of the health and fitness industry tends to ignore the simple in favor of the expensive and elite.

For the average person, barriers to entry and the wide world of health and fitness often translate into an inactive lifestyle. Combine this with a nine-to-five office job devoid of physical activity, and you're most likely living an almost completely sedentary lifestyle. A consistently sedentary lifestyle for many years can have drastic impacts on all facets of your life, from your career to your interpersonal relationships. Before we get to all of that though, let's ask a simple question —What are the risks of a sedentary life?

WALKING IMPROVES YOUR PHYSICAL HEALTH

According to the U.S. National Library of Medicine, a sedentary lifestyle can simply be defined by two factors: a lack of moderate-intensity activity and a daily routine dominated by sitting and lying down ("Health Risks of an," n.d.). This definition casts a relatively wide net, I know. In theory, this could potentially apply to everyone with a traditional nine-to-five office job, and even a large portion of the world's aging population. To narrow down the definition a bit more, the Mayo Clinic states that 30 minutes of moderate physical activity per day makes a person's lifestyle more in line with a generally "good" lifestyle (Laskowski, 2021). If you're seeking to lose weight or focus on training a specific part of your body, however, you'll need to spend more than 30 minutes per day exercising. If this goal sounds difficult, know that you're not alone. The same resource from the National Library of Medicine states the United States (along with many other countries around the world) is spending increasingly more time sitting and lying down. Our culture is largely one of work productivity, and sitting down at an office job for most of the day doesn't bode well for our physical (or mental) health. A 2022 report published by the U.S. Centers for Disease Control and Prevention states that a whopping 25% of all Americans are "physically inactive," with states like West Virginia, Oklahoma, Louisiana, Alabama, Kentucky, Arkansas, and Mississippi all reporting an inactivity rate of 30% or higher (Ali, 2022). In short, while you are ultimately responsible for your own health, it's an undeniable fact that we all live in a largely unhealthy society.

Unfortunately, these numbers have very real effects on people's quality of life. According to Dietician Sneha Jain (n.d.), a sedentary lifestyle can manifest itself through a variety of negative factors such as:

- poor digestion and constipation
- stiff joints
- puffy eyes and facial features
- persistent feelings of tiredness or fatigue
- weight changes
- poor or decreased sleep
- worsening preexisting health factors
- sugar, salt, alcohol, or substance cravings

…and much more.

While each of these symptoms is bad enough on its own, a chronically inactive lifestyle can result in compounding problems. In other words, these symptoms, continuing over a long period of time and increasing in intensity can sometimes cause irreversible damage to your physical and mental health. More specifically, worsening preexisting conditions, cardiovascular issues, and mental health deterioration are sometimes precursors to even bigger medical and mental conditions, including (but most certainly not limited to):

- **Obesity**

As you likely already know, obesity is a condition in which your body accumulates much more fat than it needs. In terms of actual numbers, The World Health Organization categorizes any body mass index (BMI) over 25 as "overweight," and any BMI over 30 as "obese" ("Obesity," 2020). This might sound innocuous at first, but carrying around more weight than your body needs is a major contributor to quickly deteriorating health. According to the Harvard School of Public Health, obesity and excess weight, "diminishes almost every aspect of health, from reproductive and respiratory function to memory and mood" ("Health Risks | Obesity," 2012).

How does excess weight make all of this happen, though? Think of it this way—If you're a server in a restaurant, your job is going to be more difficult if the place is packed to the brim with guests. Your body is made up of many different parts (the servers of your restaurant, so to speak). While each part has its own job, it's still impacted by the state of the system as a whole. When a person is medically obese, all of the individual parts of their body have to work extra hard to accommodate the excess fat. Since all of the different parts of your body are connected, one small change can upset how your entire system works. The best way to combat obesity is (you guessed it!) an active lifestyle.

- **Heart disease**

Unlike other conditions related to an inactive lifestyle, heart disease can actually refer to several different illnesses. The broader categorization of heart disease can mean anything from coronary artery disease, to chronic arrhythmias, to heart valve diseases like endocarditis and rheumatic heart disease. In short, there are many things that can potentially injure your heart and all of its complex inner workings. Heart disease and other related risk factors can also cause medical emergencies like heart attacks, strokes, and even heart failure. The best way to get your heart in good working order is to use it—walking, even for a few minutes per day, is always a good idea. In the long term, your heart will thank you ("About Heart Disease," 2019)!

- **High blood pressure**

High blood pressure, also called hypertension, occurs when the blood inside your body puts excess pressure on the walls of your arteries. This can happen for multiple reasons (like genetics and stress), but hypertension is also a sign of unhealthy habits and conditions like obesity, diet, smoking or substance use, and lack of exercise. High blood pressure often accompanies heart disease and a leading contributor to heart attacks, strokes, and heart failure (Jaret, 2021). One of the best ways to prevent hypertension, along with dietary adjustments and substance use cessation, is consistent aerobic workouts. In other words: Exercise! While we'll discuss aerobic workouts in more detail later, aerobic exercise can include any activity that elevates your heart rate for an extended period of time. For the purposes of building a sustainable workout routine, brisk walking can also constitute a form of aerobic exercise.

- **High cholesterol**

Cholesterol, a waxy element in your blood, comes in two forms—low-density lipoprotein (LDL) and high-density lipoprotein (HDL). In general, LDL is the worse of the two. HDL, on the other hand, actually picks up LDL and carries it away to your liver, where it is then broken down and expelled out of your body. While this waxy substance keeps your body healthy and strong when it's at the proper levels, too much cholesterol of either variety can have negative (and serious!) effects on your cardiovascular health. As it builds in your blood, high cholesterol levels (specifically LDL) may eventually result in narrowing arteries, which in turn increases your blood pressure. Unfortunately, unlike other conditions associated with a sedentary lifestyle, high cholesterol levels don't come with any warning signs. Rather, your doctor or primary care physician must run blood tests in order to determine your cholesterol levels. In other words, you may not be aware that you're at risk until you start experiencing conditions such as high blood pressure, obesity, or heart disease. Lack of exercise lowers the level of HDL in your blood, which means that your arteries aren't getting cleaned of bad cholesterol. The good news is that a lifestyle with just 60 minutes of exercise per week, or less than 10 minutes of exercise per day, can increase your HDL levels, according to the Mayo Clinic (Mayo Clinic Staff, 2022b).

- **Metabolic syndrome**

If all of the conditions we've discussed so far weren't bad enough on their own, Metabolic syndrome is often used to describe two or more of these conditions in a person. The term "metabolic syndrome" can be used to describe anyone with a combination of hypertension, high blood sugar, obesity, and high cholesterol. Being diagnosed with metabolic syndrome is unfortunately common in the United States, with an estimated one-third of American adults diagnosed ("Metabolic Syndrome," 2021). Metabolic syndrome, along with the symptoms that accompany the conditions it describes, also puts you at a much higher risk for developing type 2 diabetes and chronic heart disease.

- **Type 2 diabetes**

While diabetes is commonly associated with a poor diet, a sedentary and inactive lifestyle can also contribute to the progression of the condition. Generally, type 2 diabetes can be attributed to two physiological factors. Firstly, your pancreas doesn't produce enough insulin, a hormone that breaks down sugar. Secondly, your cells don't take in as much sugar as they should. These two things result in an excess of sugar in the bloodstream, which gets worse when you maintain a poor or sugar-heavy diet. While diet is indeed important, your activity levels also play a major role in the development of diabetes.

Don't worry, you don't need to be a chemist or a biologist to understand how type 2 diabetes works! Let's break it down—essentially, when you're not moving, your body stores up sugar from the food you've eaten in the form of glucose. Your body will later use that glucose when it needs energy, namely when you're exercising. When there's too much sugar in your bloodstream, and your body isn't using the glucose it's already stored, your pancreas gets overloaded and can't produce enough insulin to break everything down. While it can certainly be managed and improved with consistent exercise and a good diet, type 2 diabetes can't be cured ("Metabolic Syndrome," 2021).

- **Cancer**

According to the Australian-based charity Cancer Council, a lack of daily physical activity causes an approximated 11% of breast cancer cases after menopause and 14% of colon cancer cases ("Move Your Body," n.d.). Unfortunately, your risk of cancer isn't limited to colon and breast cancers—prostate, uterine, and lung cancers are also likely for those who live mainly sedentary lifestyles. Like the Mayo Clinic, Cancer Council also recommends a minimum of 30 minutes of exercise per day, on as many days of the week as you can manage. An estimated 60 minutes of exercise per day can drastically decrease your chances of developing cancer; and fortunately, you can also split your daily workouts into smaller segments of twenty (or even ten) minutes ("Move Your Body," n.d.). The more activity, the better!

- **Osteoporosis**

Osteoporosis is a condition that affects the strength of your bones, making them more brittle and prone to fractures and breaks. While anyone can potentially develop osteoporosis, older folks are generally more at risk. Like high cholesterol, osteoporosis doesn't have any apparent symptoms associated with it, and you can potentially go for years without recognizing the condition. For many, osteoporosis manifests in hip breaks or fractures, spinal injuries, and wrist break following a fall. Along with a diet that includes a steady stream of calcium and vitamin D, getting active can also lessen your chances of developing osteoporosis. Like any muscle or strength training, maintaining bone strength and mass starts with using that part of your body, preferably through weight-bearing activities (like walking!) (Garrick, 2017).

With all of the aforementioned risks in mind, let's examine what this means for everyday people who live sedentary lifestyles. According to one 2020 study from a team of Korean researchers, nearly one-third of the global population aged 15 and older don't exercise enough to be sufficiently healthy (Park et al., 2020). For America, this means that 8.3% of annual deaths are attributed to a sedentary lifestyle, according to the CDC (Carlson et al., 2018). In a nation of 333.3 million at the time of this writing ("U.S. and World," 2022), this means that nearly 28 million people die from complications of inactivity *per year*. This is especially tragic knowing that most of these untimely deaths are preventable.

And as if all of these physical symptoms weren't enough, your mental health can also be strongly impacted by your lifestyle choices.

WALKING IMPROVES YOUR MENTAL HEALTH

As you might have guessed, health experts and physicians generally agree that there is an unavoidable connection between your physical and mental health. This wasn't always the case, however. Traditional healing practices outside of the broader West, like those in Asia and the Indigenous Americas, usually included a variety of methods that took care of both the body and mind. On the other hand, the West had separated the body and mind into two distinct parts by the 16th century, in large part due to philosophers and scholars like Descartes and Sir Isaac Newton. According to Descartes' concept of Reductionism, the human body (and by extension, the universe) operated as a complex machine might operate, with each individual part serving a broader purpose by doing its job. Descartes believed that the mind was only a small, albeit important, part of the human machine. The goal of our human machine, according to him, was to keep the body in good, functioning order. As you might imagine, this idea of Reductionism began a centuries-long Western tradition of mind-body separatism and indifference to one's mental well-being (Massey, 2015).

Today, Western medicine is (fortunately) in a very different place, in large part due to discoveries like the placebo effect during the Second World War. In today's world, the mind-body connection (sometimes called mind-body modality) is still in the process of making its way into the mainstream. If you've been on Instagram, or any social media platform in recent years, you've likely seen a big uptick in the amount of content relating to "self-care." Although it's not exactly thought about in these terms, self-care can be a great way to recognize the connection between mental and physical health.

How does all of this relate to walking, you may wonder? Well, as you know, walking is an easy way of integrating physical activity into your daily life. By extension, an increase in walking can have very noticeable effects on your mood, social interactions, and broader mental health. In fact, according to many sources, a sedentary lifestyle without much walking or other physical exercise is likely to manifest many negative mental and cognitive symptoms. For former athletes and older folks, this can appear as forgetting things more easily, struggling with otherwise basic daily tasks, or even feelings of inadequacy. For many, regardless of age, a sedentary life can also result in drastic changes in mood and mental conditions such as increased anxiety or feelings of depression.

Circling back to the dietary expertise of Sneha Jain, consistent or long-term inactivity can result in the following mental symptoms:

- worsening memory
- poor concentration
- increased anxiety
- feelings of sadness or a progressively worsening mood

All of these symptoms, both cognitive and emotional, are actually due to a neurological process that occurs after prolonged inactivity. That's correct—a primarily sedentary lifestyle can actually change your brain chemistry! Unfortunately, beginning a sustainable and long-term exercise routine becomes much more difficult when your own brain is fighting against you. Conversely, when you are consistently physically active, your body responds by releasing beneficial neurochemicals like serotonin. Serotonin, sometimes called a "feel-good" chemical, is responsible for a wide range of processes like mood, digestion, wound healing, bone mass, sleep patterns, blood clotting, memory, body temperature, hunger, and even libido. As a neurotransmitter, serotonin acts as a messenger between your brain and your body. Consequently, when this messenger becomes unbalanced, your body may misinterpret (or miss entirely) the natural signals that your brain is sending out. This can result in an array of mental and cognitive symptoms, including memory trouble, mood swings, and poor sleep. An approximated 90% of your body's serotonin lives in your gut, with the remaining serotonin living in and around your brain. Exercise, even in small doses, encourages these serotonin deposits to move and circulate, effectively strengthening the connection between the body and the brain.

A lack of serotonin, as is common in people who live a more sedentary lifestyle, is usually attached to conditions like chronic depression, anxiety, mania, PTSD, panic disorders, schizophrenia, and other psychological conditions ("Serotonin: What is it," n.d.). Let's be clear—serious mental conditions like depression and anxiety are oftentimes extremely complex. If you've ever experienced major depression or similar conditions, you're likely aware that simply going for a run isn't going to cure you of your mental symptoms. That being said, being consistently active may decrease some of the symptoms you experience—or even the severity of your symptoms overall. While consistently walking once per day is not a cure-all, it can greatly contribute to an overall better mood in the long term.

Additionally, there's a wider societal and cultural element to inactivity and its associated symptoms, namely obesity. Even if you don't take part in social media, there is a very strong message that communication channels like movies, shows, and advertising send out to the broader American audience: In short, obesity is something to avoid at all costs. This message, as you'll notice, says absolutely nothing about physical or mental health, instead placing importance on societal aesthetics. Aversion to obesity, regardless of health, has disastrous consequences for those who are just beginning their fitness journey. According to one study described in *Yes! Magazine*, just 15% of hiring managers would consider hiring an overweight woman. Another study from the same article states that obese employees are both hired and compensated considerably less than their thinner counterparts (Feder, 2019). This is unfortunately just one piece of a larger puzzle. The "fat tax," as it's often called, describes the economic, cultural, and interpersonal consequences of fatphobia. This social conditioning can start as early as the age of three, and one 2008 study from the University of

Central Florida even found that nearly half of American girls from the ages of three to six were worried about being perceived as fat (Hayes, 2004). To make matters worse, low-income people and families are generally more at risk for inactivity and obesity, with women of all races being notably more prone to developing obesity while in a low-income situation (Zare et al., 2021).

Though health is certainly important, social messaging toward those who lead more sedentary lives can have a massive negative impact on those who are obese or overweight. Guilt, shame, or otherwise negative or self-deprecating feelings ultimately *do not* help people lose weight or live more active lifestyles. This broader societal messaging has the potential to significantly impact those with preexisting mental conditions like anxiety or depression, making the journey toward optimum health even more difficult.

With this in mind, it's important to acknowledge the challenges that may lie ahead of you in your fitness journey. Your goals, whatever they are, should revolve first and foremost around improving your own physical and mental health. If you approach your physical health from a place of self-care and kindness, you'll find that your fitness will be far more sustainable than it would be otherwise. In other words—don't be hard on yourself! The first step, no matter how small, has the potential to change your health (and life) for the better.

DETERMINING YOUR BASELINE CONDITION

In the spirit of self-care and kindness, let us begin by meeting ourselves where we are on the journey. Going on a brisk walk is all well and good, but building a sustainable, long-term fitness routine is a bit deeper than that. If you want to see results over time, you need to know where you are beginning. So before you go out and buy an expensive scale or fancy workout equipment, stop for a moment and consider—just like walking, you can easily measure your progress without the help of the fitness industry. It's also worth noting that a scale isn't the best measure of one's health. Your weight doesn't communicate anything about your body composition, for example, nor does it take into consideration anything else that might be going on inside your body. If your biggest health goal is to lose weight, then you might want to invest in a good scale; but for many, seeing a number on a scale can actually be counterproductive. For those who aren't purchasing extra equipment, all you'll need is a watch, a big space you can easily move around in, and an open (and kind!) mindset. In general, there are five aspects of your bodily health that you should be aware of: upper body, lower body, core, flexibility, and endurance. Most at-home fitness tests will test the first three categories (upper body, lower body, and core) for strength. Flexibility tests aren't usually separated by region, but you'll find that most of the focus on flexibility falls on your lower body and back. Finally, endurance measures how fast you tire during exercise, and is a generally good indicator of cardiovascular health. While it might not seem like it at first glance, walking consistently can actually impact all of these areas in a big way, increasing overall strength, cardiovascular endurance, and flexibility.

Of course, your fitness journey and the goals you set depend on you. The fitness tests we are about to cover are a good place to start, there is also a wide variety of fitness tests that can be found online. Additionally, you may also decide that you want to focus on a particular part of your bodily health and ignore the other tests. No matter what you decide, it may be helpful to have a basic knowledge of fitness testing in case you decide to start measuring yourself in the future.

Upper Body Testing

Upper body tests usually focus on push-ups, although there are several variations of push-up tests. If you can do a push-up with your legs fully extended, great! If you're not there yet, you can certainly test with your knees on the floor. In terms of proper form, you always want your back to be as straight as possible, tucking in your tailbone as you move. You also want to make sure that your arms are reaching a proper 90° angle when you dip, so that your humerus (the bone in your arm connecting your shoulder and your elbow) is parallel to the ground and flush with the side of your body. When you begin with arms fully extended, then lowered to 90°, and back up again, this counts as one repetition. This is the number you want to keep track of, either in a physical journal or digitally.

The testing process itself is simple—do as many push-ups as you can without breaking proper form. After recording your repetitions, hold onto your results for future reference. If you like, you can also research push-up fitness test charts online, which outline one's upper body strength level through brackets. Most of these charts look something like this one from Verywell Fit (Quinn, 2020):

	Age 20-29	Age 30-39	Age 40-49	Age 50-59	Age 60+
Excellent	48+	39+	34+	29+	19+
Good	34-48	25-39	20-34	15-29	5-19
Average	17-33	12-24	8-19	6-14	3-4
Poor	6-16	4-11	3-7	2-5	1-2
Very poor	6 or less	4 or less	3 or less	2 or less	1 or less

If you decide to measure yourself based on charts like this one, it's important to consider both your age and the sex you were assigned at birth. Most of the time, push-up testing charts for males include more repetitions than those for women; and as you can see from the chart above, older folks will almost always include fewer repetitions.

Core Strength Testing

Core testing, sometimes also called stability testing, measures both your core strength and some upper body strength. Usually, core strength tests will have you hold a plank position, like what you might see when you start a push-up with your toes on the ground. Historically, core tests included activities like crunches and sit-ups, but these exercises usually aren't the best indicator of core strength.

The test itself is even more simple than the push-up test. If you can hold a plank for 60 seconds or more, you're considered to have excellent core strength. For most, the average hold time for a plank is 30-60 seconds. According to SPOTEBI Fitness and Nutrition, if you can not hold a plank position for 30 seconds or more, you're generally considered to have relatively poor core strength ("At-Home Fitness," 2021).

Lower Body Testing

Lower body strength is usually measured by bodyweight squats, although you may see some lower body tests include things like calf raises, hurdle jumps, steps, or wall squats. For our purposes, however, bodyweight squats are especially beneficial. In addition to helping you develop the habit of good posture, bodyweight squats are also simple, easy to measure in repetitions, and don't require any equipment. Proper posture for a bodyweight squat starts with having your feet shoulder-width apart from each other and squatting until your hips reach the level of your knees (or until your thighs are parallel to the floor). Starting from a standing position, bending your knees, and then extending them fully is considered one repetition.

Unlike upper body and core strength testing, it's a good idea to have a stopwatch handy for this test. Usually, your lower body is stronger than your upper body, so waiting until you tire yourself out with squats might take awhile. Instead, time yourself for one minute, and see how many squats you can do while maintaining the correct form. As with upper body testing, there are several charts online that can tell you a bit more about your results. As a general baseline, check out this chart from SPOTEBI Fitness and Nutrition ("At-Home Fitness," 2021):

	Age 20-29	Age 30-39	Age 40-49	Age 50-59	Age 60+
Excellent	29+	26+	23+	20+	17+
Good	24-28	21-25	18-22	15-19	12-16
Average	21-23	18-20	15-17	12-14	9-11
Poor	19-20	16-17	13-14	10-11	7-8
Very poor	<18	<15	<12	<9	<6

With this exercise in particular, it might be easier to count your repetitions while you stand in front of a mirror so that you can see your form. Alternatively, you can also have a friend or family member count your repetitions and view your form for you.

Flexibility Testing

While full-body flexibility is certainly important for your health, back and lower body flexibility is especially important. This is especially true if you're planning on sticking to a new aerobic exercise regimen—like walking for 30 minutes every day! The easiest way to measure back and lower body flexibility is through the "box" exercise. This exercise requires a few extra pieces of equipment—namely a box of some kind, a ruler, and some tape.

To do this exercise, sit flat on the floor with your legs fully extended, placing the soles of your feet against the outside of the box. Before you start, tape the ruler to the top of the box, lining up the end of the ruler with the edge of the box. Now, simply reach toward your toes, stretching as far as you can past the edge of the top of the box. At your biggest stretch, look at where your fingers are on the ruler. After stretching as far as you comfortably can, make a note of how many inches or centimeters you were able to reach on the ruler. Again, you might need help from another person to see how many inches you were able to reach. According to SPOTEBI Fitness and Nutrition, anywhere from 0.5 to 4 inches is average for all ages, with 8 inches or more considered excellent flexibility ("At-Home Fitness," 2021).

Endurance Testing

Depending on which endurance test you choose, you may need to revisit some basic algebra skills. Don't worry! We'll walk through the basics together.

There are a wide range of endurance testing exercises out there, so you may want to do some additional research to find out what test will work best for you. To give you an idea of what an endurance test entails, let's go over the Cooper test. The Cooper test, once used by the American military in the 1960s, is a good standard to see how efficiently your body uses oxygen during aerobic exercise (otherwise known as your VO2 max). The more efficiently you use oxygen while you run, the further you'll be able to run within a given time. For instance, someone with a VO2 max of 30 is going to run further in 12 minutes than someone with a VO2 max of 25. The test, conducted over a period of 12 minutes, only requires one piece of information—how far you were able to run, in kilometers. After you run for 12 minutes and determine your distance, you then plug the distance (D) into the following formula:

$$VO2\,Max = (22.351\,D) - 11.288$$

So, say you were able to run 2 kilometers in 12 minutes. Plugging this into the equation, you'd get something that looks a little like this:

$$VO2\,Max = (22.351\,\cdot 2) - 11.288$$
Thus: $VO2\,Max = 44.702 - 11.288$
And your result is: $VO2\,Max = 33.414$

Once you know your VO2 max, you can search online for VO2 max charts to see where you fall based on your age group and gender. According to Verywell Fit, the average man will have a VO2 max value somewhere around 35 or 40 mL/kg/min, while the average woman will have a VO2 max value somewhere around 30 mL/kg/min (Quinn, 2022). By this standard, the example VO2 max that we found using the formula is above average for women and below average for men. However, you should also keep in mind that there are several other factors that might impact your score, like age and the altitude in which you are running. If you don't feel like using a formula at all, there are also some online VO2 max calculators that will tell you what your scores mean, such as the 12-minute run calculator on ExRx.net. Additionally, if the Cooper test doesn't sound like what you're looking for, there are also tests like the Pacer that might work better for your situation or space.

Establishing a baseline for your body can be daunting for people of all ages, genders, and backgrounds. That being said, it's important to treat yourself well throughout this process. Meeting yourself where you currently are on your fitness journey is the first step toward improving your quality of life, and you'll likely find that the first step is the most intimidating. Regardless of societal standards, guilt, or other pressures you might face, keep in mind that your health (mental and physical) is the only thing that truly matters. Once you have a baseline for your body, it's time to move on to the easy (and fun) part—Walking!

In the next chapter, we'll move through some changes and improvements you might see as a result of your walking routine, as well as some things to keep in mind throughout the process.

2

WALK AWAY YOUR WORRIES

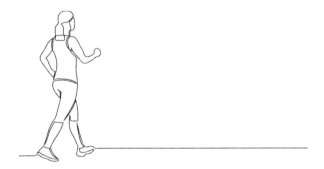

> *If you are in a bad mood, go for a walk. If you are still in a bad mood, go for another walk.*
>
> — HIPPOCRATES

At this point, we know that a sedentary lifestyle can hurt our health over time. Obesity, heart conditions, diabetes, and poor mental health stem from too much inactivity, and most of these conditions are avoidable with consistent exercise. But how much of an impact does a 15-minute morning walk have, really? Oddly enough, Hippocrates (often referred to as the father of western medicine) *loved* to prescribe walking. Bad day? Take a walk. Stress at work? Take a walk. Existential crisis? Take a very, very long walk. In a Western world full of pharmacological antidotes for nearly every ailment that one might experience, however, the father of western medicine seems largely ignored. How this dissonance arose is a matter of debate, but one thing is certain—just *taking a walk* is relatively uncommon nowadays. According to The Institute for Transportation and Development Policy, cities in the United States are far less walkable than many of their international counterparts (Teale, 2020), in large part due to high levels of pedestrian deaths, urban sprawl, and failing to include pedestrian infrastructure like sidewalks or crosswalks. If you live outside of an urban or suburban area, you probably live in an even less walkable area. Rural folks, perhaps even more so than city dwellers, rely on personal vehicles like cars as their only form of transportation. In a system like this, considering that the vast majority of people—an estimated 80%, more specifically—have sedentary day jobs, it's no wonder that Hippocrates has taken a back seat (Gremaud et al., 2018).

However, all is not lost. Walking—no matter where, no matter when—still counts! Walking from one room to another multiple times a day counts as walking, walking to your coworker's cubicle to ask them a question counts as walking, and even walking to your kitchen for breakfast every morning counts as walking. Every step that you take during your day is a step toward better health outcomes, quite literally. In fact, one group of researchers from Oregon State University determined that light exercise, like normal walking that you might do to move from one room to another, could potentially be just as effective as more high-intensity exercise, especially for older adults (Bergland, 2015). The main takeaway here is that all movement, no matter how small, *can and will* make a difference in your quality of life.

The benefits that you see from daily movement range from small and short-term (like calming acute anxiety), or big and long-term (like reducing your risk of developing cancer). If you don't believe me, take it from the experts:

According to the American Psychological Association, walking (even less than the daily recommended amount) can reduce symptoms of depression by up to 18% compared to those who don't walk at all. Those who did meet the daily recommendations for walking saw a whopping 25% decrease in their symptoms of depression. The same 2022 study found that 1 in 9 cases of medically-diagnosed depression in the United States could be prevented by following CDC guidelines for exercise (DeAngelis, 2022). In short, if you're experiencing feelings of chronic depression, you might find that walking minimizes your symptoms.

According to a study from a group of Stanford researchers, those who participate in 90-minute outdoor walks show notably decreased levels of rumination (Bratman et al., 2015). Rumination, a symptom often associated with depression, happens when a thought or series of thoughts get caught in a loop in your mind, and these thoughts often revolve around dark or sad subjects. Physically, these negative mind loops often show up as neurological activity in a part of your brain called the prefrontal cortex. The prefrontal cortex, which doesn't develop until you reach 25 (coincidentally why you're not allowed to rent a car until you're older), is primarily responsible for long-term concepts and problems. This can manifest through a number of things such as behavior, inhibitions, planning, problem-solving, memory, intelligence, language, and even vision and eye movements. Additionally, a damaged or dysfunctional prefrontal cortex has also been linked to conditions like medically significant apathy, depression, schizophrenia, mania, depression, and even dementia (Siddiqui et al., 2008). In other words, the Stanford researchers found that there was a decreased stimulation of the subgenual prefrontal cortex in the study participants, effectively changing their neurochemistry for the better as they walked through the natural environment.

A 2014 study conducted by a different group of Stanford researchers found that walking, regardless of location or scenery, notably increased the participants' creative thinking (Oppezzo & Schwartz, 2014). More specifically, walking was empirically shown to increase analogical creativity, novel ideas, and ideation more generally. Whether or not you define yourself as a creative person, the ability to develop new ideas in different areas of your life (and analogical creativity specifically) is an extremely important skill in your career, interpersonal relationships, and mental health. What does this mean in practice, however? Well, once you start looking for them, you'll quickly realize that analogies are a big part of how we interact with the world—by comparing two similar subjects, we're able to make connections between subjects that would otherwise be unrelated. This can happen with nearly every facet of our lives, from physical objects to spaces and social situations—and analogical thinking is a key part of how we're able to solve problems.

In one 2016 study in Japan, researchers found that participants' sleep duration, quality, and latency were improved by walking every day (Hori et al., 2016). Sleep duration, as you might've guessed, refers to how long you sleep each night. How long you sleep each night is certainly an important factor—I don't know about you, but I've been told countless times that I should ideally get somewhere between seven and nine hours of sleep per night. That being said, the quantity of your sleep might not mean that much if the quality of your sleep isn't good. Sleep can be broadly broken down into four stages, all of which are important to the quality of your dozing. That being said, deep sleep and rapid eye movement (REM) sleep are especially important for things like memory consolidation, learning, emotional processing, metabolic balancing, immune functions, and dreaming. Generally, it's recommended that you should get about an hour or two of deep sleep per night, and about two hours of REM sleep per night. Without these two stages of sleep, you might find that you're more irritable, less focused, and more forgetful. In the same vein, sleep disturbances will interrupt these crucial stages of sleep more often than not, leading to noticeable signs of sleep deprivation. As the Japanese team discovered, participants who walked every day for at least four weeks saw a significant difference in both the amount of sleep they got each night, as well as the number of sleep disturbances that they encountered (Hori et al., 2016).

Lack of sleep and poor sleep quality aren't the only problems that can arise during bedtime, however. If you struggle with tossing and turning when you try to go to bed, this one's for you. Sleep latency, or the amount of time that it takes you to fall asleep, can be one of the key factors in chronic insomnia. According to The Pittsburgh Sleep Quality Index (PSQI) used by the Japanese researchers, study participants with sleep latency issues saw drastically improved sleep latency times when they took daily walks. More specifically, participants who led more sedentary lives reported an even bigger improvement in sleep latency than participants who were already active (Hori et al., 2016). In other words, those who might be struggling with sleep issues due to inactivity or associated conditions will likely find that they fall asleep much faster when they walk every day.

While the benefits of daily movement are possible for everyone regardless of gender or age, older folks have the potential to see some more immediate benefits. The term "white matter" may sound like a comic book super substance from outer space, but it's actually used to describe the matter that lies deeper in your brain. This white matter is made up of nerve fibers covered in a white protective material called myelin, like a phone charger cable protected by a plastic covering. In the same way that a phone charger cable carries electricity from your wall outlet to your smartphone, the white matter in your brain is responsible for sending electrical signals to different parts of your body—this effectively determines what you think, feel, and do. As you age, this white matter (and all of the very important parts that it contains) tends to deteriorate—blood flow to the white matter decreases, the myelin sheaths surrounding your nerve fibers begin to weaken, and the electrical signals carrying important information may get lost. As a result, older folks are more prone to conditions like chronic white matter disease, which can mean changes in balance, walking, basic physical functions, cognition, and memory issues. Alzheimer's disease is usually associated with white matter deterioration, which can be especially scary if you're genetically prone to the condition ("White Matter Disease," n.d.).

Oddly enough, white matter disease is very strongly connected to another set of conditions that we've already talked about. Metabolic disease and white matter disease go hand in hand, namely because white matter disease is significantly worsened by cardiovascular illnesses and poor blood flow. If only there was a way that you could prevent both conditions at the same time... Wait! As it turns out, a study published in the science journal *NeuroImage* found that white matter plasticity (or the proper functioning of all your different neurological parts) is greatly improved with consistent aerobic exercise. The study, while also including activities like dancing and yoga, named walking as one of the most impactful activities on participants' white matter plasticity, with participants walking anywhere from 20 to 40 minutes every day for six weeks. Through neurological imaging techniques and a series of cognitive tests, the researchers concluded that adopting a daily walking routine meant that, "white matter in the adult brain retains plasticity in vulnerable regions and that these changes can be observed on a short-term scale" (Mendez Colmenares et al., 2021).

White matter plasticity is just one piece of a larger physiological and psychological picture—a longer and higher quality life. You already know a bit about quality improvement from our discussion in the last chapter, but we haven't yet talked about longevity as a whole. Luckily, there are still more handy research studies to help us better understand the benefits of daily activity. One of these studies, published in the British Journal of Sports Medicine in 2019, discovered that people who exercised for 10 to 60 minutes per week saw a nearly 20% decreased risk of death compared to those who did not (Rabbitt, 2022). The same study also showed that the gap grows when you comply with recommended activity guidelines, with the risk of death decreasing by 31%. So the early walking prescription advice from Hippocrates holds up just as well today!

OTHER SURPRISING BENEFITS OF WALKING

Aside from the basic benefits of living longer, losing weight, sleeping well, and keeping yourself happy and healthy, there are also some unconventional benefits that you might not have anticipated. For one, walking every day can actually help those with a sweet tooth (or sweet teeth, in my case). Two research studies from the University of Exeter determined that just a 15-minute walk can help you lose cravings for sweets and snacks, even when the food you want is right in front of you. A similar 2015 study drew the same conclusion, adding that exercise doesn't even have to happen consistently for your sweet tooth to fall out (Ledochowski et al., 2015). A one-time 15-minute walk, in addition to burning calories and getting you moving, can also decrease your sugar intake. That sounds like a win-win to me!

In addition to physical benefits, getting outside for a quick walk can also do wonders for your social and professional life. Perhaps the greatest thing about walking as an exercise is that it's extremely versatile—if you feel the need to multitask, walking is a great opportunity to check many things off of your to-do list. For instance, daily walks can help you:

- **Learn a new skill**

Technology is a wonderful thing. If you have a smart device and some headphones, you're all set to turn your daily walk into a reading or learning session. From audiobooks to podcasts to webinars, there is basically no limit to the things that you can listen to while you move around. If you've been hoping to find time to reread some classics, now is your chance! If you want to invest in a new career skill, language, or hobby, there is a world of different podcasts out there to fit your every need. Services like Spotify, Apple Music, and Libby are excellent options if you want to grow your mind while improving your physical health.

- **Improve Communication and Collaboration**

Walking is a perfect time to catch up on missed calls with family, friends and colleagues. Walking in a park or outdoor area can provide a relaxed and informal setting for conversation, collaboration, and creative problem-solving. When with another person, walking side-by-side provides opportunities for one-on-one conversations and allows for more personal connections to be formed. You may also choose to walk with a group, which can help build stronger relationships and foster a sense of community.

- **Get in your "me" time**

Living with family or a roommate, while lovely, can sometimes be a little overwhelming. Part of self-care and mental health maintenance is knowing where and when to draw your boundaries, and walking can help in doing so. Getting out for your daily walk can give you a chance to catch your breath, manage and process your emotions, and take a break from stressful cohabitation. Simply pop in your headphones, turn on some music, and open your front door.

- **Enjoy complementary outdoor activities**

Walking can open up a whole new world of outdoor activities that you may love. From bird-watching to learning about your area's local horticulture, there are loads of activities that you can do (even while you're walking!). Personally, I've found that walking, plant identification, and foraging go hand in hand—as long as you follow the proper safety requirements. In addition to contributing to my physical and mental health, I can come back from my daily walks with a natural snack!

- **Exercise your pet**

Sometimes, pets have a funny way of telling us what we need. Taking care of another animal is illuminating in many ways, and oftentimes you'll find that you share many of the same needs as your pet. If your dog has been sitting by the door and whining all day, it might be a sign that both of you need to get outside for a quick walk around the block. In addition to keeping you happy and healthy, you're also keeping your furry companion in good spirits.

- **Beat your afternoon slump**

With so many people working from home nowadays, it can be even more difficult than normal to stay motivated and attentive. When your pantry is close by, you might be tempted to reach for a bag of chips or a candy bar during your workday. On the other hand, working remotely also offers the unique benefit of being able to stand up from your workspace and change your scenery completely. That afternoon slump that you face on weekdays can be easily overcome with a good pair of walking shoes and a spare 15 minutes—and it may even make you feel more productive and creative as a result.

- **Improve your balance**

There is no doubt that as we age, our ability to maintain balance diminishes. Changes in our inner ear and overall strength may contribute to increased falls and insecure steps. One way to improve this skill is by simply practicing. One day during a walk, I challenged myself to walk the straight line of a pavement seam. It was more difficult to do than I thought! I began incorporating this exercise at the end of each walk, increasing the length of the balance exercise and eventually moving up to the "balance beam". The balance beam is basically my fun word for curb. This is a more advanced exercise of walking along the length of a raised curb which is more challenging. While these are wonderfully helpful exercises, please use caution with your surroundings and a sure footing to prevent injury.

- **Use technology to make life easier**

If you haven't yet mastered the personal assistant feature of your smart phone, you are missing out on a powerful tool. With simple verbal requests, "Personal assistants" such as *Siri, Google Assistant,* and *Alexa* are always ready to help conduct research, make shopping lists, find recipes, take notes, and text contacts. I often use my walking time to create to-do lists, plan meals, and add appointments and reminders to my calendar, all hands-free. *Siri* also helps me keep track of concepts while I brainstorm so I never forget an idea!

So far we've mostly focused on the individual rewards of a daily walking routine. Personal benefits aren't something to be understated, but social and cultural advantages are also important to discuss (especially as it pertains to mental health and community). Although you can certainly walk by yourself, it may fit your situation better if you walk with a friend or a group. In addition to holding you accountable for your new daily routine, this can also serve as an investment into your personal relationships. Catching up with friends doesn't necessarily need to happen over a glass of wine, and exercise has the potential to be a bonding exercise. Walking in a group is a great way to hold yourself accountable, while also sharing tips, ideas, and resources for your new lifestyle.

With regard to community-based benefits, there are several ways in which walking can be better than driving. It may be a little difficult to see your individual impact in a community, so let me give you a few examples. Given that only about 12% of Americans remain in their hometown for their entire life ("Do Most Americans," n.d.), chances are that you've moved to a different area of the country at least once. From personal experience, I can say with some certainty that moving to a different area than the one you grew up in can be tough, especially if you don't identify with the culture or community as much at first. Getting outside and walking each day can actually help you get to know a new area in depth, more so than if you were to simply drive around in a car. During your walks, try to remain in the present moment, and ask yourself questions about the things that you see around you. *Is that a new storefront? Where does that path lead? What language were those passersby speaking?* In a short time, you'll know all there is to know about your area's local culture and residents.

Additionally, pedestrian traffic is a great way to support your local businesses, even if you don't make a purchase. By increasing awareness of your surroundings, you're effectively taking an active part in helping small, independently-owned businesses grow and thrive (this is especially true if you bring people along on your walks). If you enjoy people-watching or keeping up with local happenings and news, try integrating these hobbies into your physical routines. Avoiding driving will also help you support your local community—and other walking enthusiasts in your area—by normalizing pedestrian activity in the area.

Aside from meeting new people in your community and supporting local businesses, physical activity can also be a great way to help causes you care about. If you're anywhere near a city, regardless of size, you'll likely find that organizations in your area organize 5Ks, 10Ks, and marathons to show support for charities. Depending on your situation and local scenery, walking to do your daily errands is an excellent way to save on carbon emissions (and gas prices). One University of Michigan finding reported that "Every gallon of gasoline you save avoids 22 pounds of CO_2 emissions… Avoiding just 10 miles of driving every week would eliminate about 500 pounds of carbon dioxide emissions a year" ("Green Facts," n.d.). I know that 10 miles might sound like a lot of walking at first, depending on your perspective, but let me make a suggestion: Do you remember the last time you got lost in a really good story? When you were watching that one great movie, or reading that one great book and time seemed to just evaporate? I have good news—you can do the things you enjoy, like getting lost in a great book, *while you walk*. Pretty soon, you'll find that walking becomes an excellent facilitator for all the other things you enjoy in life.

At this point, I'm sure you get the idea. Naming all the benefits of daily walking is great, but facts and figures can only go so far. So, instead, let me tell you a little bit about my dog. She's a rescue mutt who absolutely adores going for walks. While otherwise usually very relaxed and somewhat standoffish, she literally spins in circles with happiness at the sight of her leash. She jumps and twists and dances around until she wears herself out, at which point I can finally put on her harness and grab the doggie bags. Some years ago, at the height of a depression resulting from the passing of my mother, walking my dog was just about the last thing on my mind. Even getting out of bed felt like a marathon.

However, one morning, my dog decided that she had finally had enough. She grabbed her harness, jumped up on the bed, and dropped it on me. It was a little assertive, sure, but she got her message across. After ignoring her for a few minutes, she started pawing at me and refused to stop, absolutely determined to get me outside. After a ridiculous amount of time spent trying to negotiate, I resigned myself to my fate—we were going on a walk. My stubborn dog decided that this was going to be a half-hour walk, and I dreaded every minute. However, when I finally persuaded her to come back to our front door, I realized that I felt more awake than I had for the entire week. Somehow the fresh air, the sight of the surrounding trees and the happy trotting of my dog had noticeably lifted my spirits. To my dog's delight, these walks became more frequent until we were walking together every day, sometimes multiple times per day. My mental health had drastically improved. In the end, all it took was a gentle (but stubborn) nudge in the right direction from a furry friend. Hippocrates would have been proud.

Unfortunately, no person (or dog) can make us do the right thing. We have to make the best decisions with the information we have, and hope that everything turns out in our favor. With that in mind, remember that it only takes 15 minutes every day for you to feel happier, healthier, and better about whatever life challenges you may be facing. Walking, and all the variation that it boasts, is perhaps the best and most accessible way to jump-start healthy habits.

In the next chapter, we'll go over some of the most basic elements of starting a walking routine, from warm-ups to pedestrian safety. Before all of that, however, we first need to look at the only piece of equipment you'll ever need—shoes!

3

FIRST STEPS

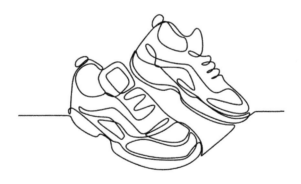

The hardest thing about exercise is to start doing it. Once you are doing exercise regularly, the hardest thing is to stop it.

— ERIN GRAY

A few weeks ago, I went out for what I thought was going to be a long walk. I had previously walked the length of the trail in question with no problems, and I had no reason to believe anything would be different this time. However, when I got to the trailhead, I quickly came to the realization that I was completely unprepared. I had failed to consider the fact that it had rained the day prior, and the entire trail was transformed into sticky, thick clay mud. As you might imagine, my poor old sneakers took a beating.

Walking as an exercise is fairly straightforward, but doing any form of exercise outdoors requires planning and preparation. For those who want to start walking every day (and possibly integrate other forms of exercise into your routine), this means investing in a pair (or multiple pairs) of good, reliable walking shoes. In turn, the shoes you choose depend on a variety of factors, like your gait, podiatric needs, and the terrain on which you walk. You never know what nature is going to throw at you, and failing to do your due diligence may lead to mud-covered sneakers and achy insoles. Even if you're not planning to walk outside, having the right sneakers for your body is crucial for preventing injury and supporting your joints properly.

Unfortunately, like the broader health and fitness industry, the world of sneakers is fraught with technical terms and various distinctions. Before you head into your local sneaker or running store, let's go over what you need to look for in a walking shoe, as well as some potential pitfalls to avoid.

SHOE SHOPPING

Let's begin by defining a few key terms that you're bound to hear in many running stores. In essence, there are only really four areas that you need to pay attention to, including:

- **Heel collar**

This is the very back of the shoe, behind your ankle. In a well-fitting shoe, the heel counter should be fairly snug, but still comfortable. If the heel collar is too loose, your foot won't be properly supported; and if the heel counter is too tight, then you'll be uncomfortable when your feet swell during your exercise.

- **Midsole**

The midsole is easily the most important component of your walking shoes, and you'll immediately notice when the midsole doesn't feel right. Sandwiched between the inside of the shoe that touches your foot and the bottom of the shoe that touches the ground, the midsole essentially makes up the structure of your shoe. Ideally, the midsole should provide support for your foot as well as shock absorption, flexibility, stability, and additional cushioning. Depending on your foot shape and walking needs, you might opt for either a thicker midsole (which is stiffer and lasts longer) or a thinner midsole (which is cushier and wears down more quickly).

- **Insole**

Attached on top of the midsole, the insole is the part of the shoe that touches your foot. The insole is much thinner than the midsole—and while it can provide some additional comfort and cushioning, it isn't the most important part of the shoe. That being said, the insole of your walking shoes should fit the sole of your feet nicely. Depending on your podiatric needs, your insole may vary with regard to the arch of your foot. Replaceable and custom insoles may also be purchased to support those with flat feet or other needs for a perfect fit.

- **Toe box**

Remember when your parents used to use a thumb to measure how well your shoes fit when you were a kid? They were onto something. The toe box (or the fabric surrounding your toes) should be tight enough to keep your foot from sliding around, but loose enough for you to be able to bend your toes. Parents typically measure this using the tried-and-true thumb test, and you can too! Well-fitting shoes should leave about a half-thumb's worth of space between your toes and the very front of the shoe.

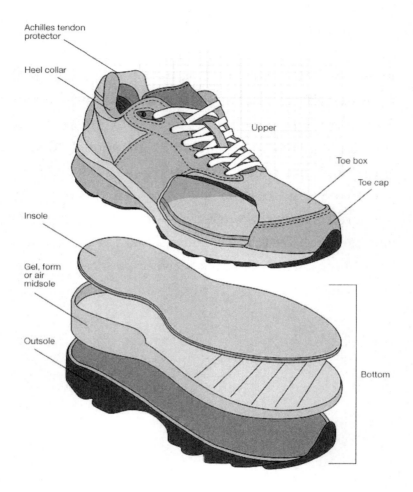

Here's where things start to get a little confusing—there is a difference between walking shoes and running shoes. While there's no hard and fast rule that says you should have different shoes for different activities, it might be a good idea to invest specifically in a pair of walking shoes. It might seem odd, but walking and running actually have several key differences when it comes to your anatomical movements. When you walk, you generally walk heel-to-toe—this means that your heel strikes the ground first, and then the rest of your foot follows. For runners, on the other hand, landing squarely on the heel of your foot would be painful, in addition to making you run slower. While running shoes require more cushioning, structure, and shock absorption, good walking shoes should instead make your step feel natural and supported. The issue here is not necessarily the differences between walking and running shoes, but rather the marketing of each. Depending on your situation, you may find a running shoe that works very well as a walking shoe, and you may also find walking shoes that don't work for you at all. In general, it may be a good idea to ignore the labels of different shoes you find. Additionally, you should know that not all big brands will work for you. Don't feel compelled to buy a pair of shoes from a well-known brand if they don't actually work with your foot.

Knowing this, you might be wondering—how should a walking shoe feel, then? In general, your ideal pair of shoes should meet four criteria:

- They feel comfortable from the moment you put them on.
- There shouldn't be too much room or too little room, and they should be sized correctly.
- Your arches should feel supported, but not suffocated.
- The shoes should have good traction on the tread (sole).

Despite knowing what you're looking for, it still may take more than a few tries before you find your perfect pair. It may help to know more about your feet and what they need before trying to purchase a pair of shoes, and this can be easily accomplished through stores that offer foot analyses. It sounds a little ridiculous, I know, but having more information might save you some serious knee pain in the long run. Personal trainers and fitness experts may also have some good information for you; and as always, you can also do your own research online if you notice a particular quality about your feet. Once you're equipped with some personalized information, it's time to find your nearest shoe store (if you haven't already).

When you have a pair of shoes in your hands, it's time to put them to the test. Before trying them on, make sure to look at the heel of the shoe. Runners require a bigger heel to prevent shock and provide stability, but walkers don't need this in a shoe. Subsequently, the height of the sole at the heel should only be about an inch taller than the height of the sole at the ball of the foot. If the heel of the shoe checks out, try twisting the shoe like you're wringing out a towel. If it's too stiff to twist with relative ease, that's not the shoe for you. You want something that's both lightweight and flexible, while still supporting your foot. While you're holding the shoe, you should also try bending the part of the shoe where the ball of your foot would sit. If it begins to bend at the arch of your foot as well, put that pair of shoes back! If, however, it's passed all of your twisting and careful assessment so far, try it on. If it's comfortable, look at the profile of the shoe in a mirror. Ideally, when you're just standing upright and still, the toe of the shoe should be raised off of the ground by a fraction of an inch.

If you find a pair of shoes you like, it might be a good idea to write it down! Unless, of course, you want to repeat the process of foot analyses and shoe shopping every year. In general, you should replace your walking shoes when you've walked about 500 miles in them according to one conclusion published in *The American Journal of Sports Medicine* (Cook et al., 2016.). That being said, every shoe is different, and so are the feet that wear them—different shoe models may need to be replaced closer to 350 miles, and your weight may also impact how fast your shoes wear out. You need to replace your shoes regularly for multiple reasons, namely because weakening support for your feet could lead to injuries. Alternatively, if you realize that you really like walking, you might also wear them until they fall apart. Once you have shoes that you're happy with, it's important to take basic care of them. This includes doing things like:

- only using your walking shoes for exercise walks
- airing out your walking shoes between uses
- washing them regularly, but not putting them in the dryer
- replacing the insoles occasionally

If you want to make your shoes last longer (or if you dread shoe shopping, like me), it may be worth it to buy two pairs of the same shoes, so that you can alternate the pairs and allow them to breathe.

Now that we have the basics out of the way, you should also know about some of the more detailed elements of shoe choice that might apply to you. I mentioned earlier that I have somewhat flat feet, and this subsequently impacts the shoes I wear when I walk. If your feet are severely flat, this is called overpronation. You may be at risk for developing joint problems, knee pain, or hip pain if you have overpronation (or the complete collapse of the arch of your foot). If you've ever had knee pain before, you know that it's no joke. If you have severely collapsed arches, you might want to look into walking shoes that offer more motion control. Motion control shoes are generally thicker and won't twist as easily, but they will offer your arch the necessary support that you need in order to be able to walk long distances. Additionally, you may also want to look into specially-made orthotic insoles that you can put into your walking shoes, which will provide more arch support. If you are obese or overweight, you may also be at risk of overpronation and knee or hip problems, so it's best to consult a professional before you buy walking shoes.

Alternatively, you can also develop underpronation, in which your body weight rolls to the outer edges of your feet, along your pinky toe. The problem with this is that when you push off the ground, your strength generally comes from your big toe. Your pinky toe isn't equipped to handle the stress of this motion, and this can also cause several posture problems. If you consistently wear shoes that don't fit your feet well, you may inadvertently cause problems like plantar fasciitis, shin splints, or even back pain.

Shoe shopping can be tedious and boring at times, but keep in mind that this investment can save you hundreds of dollars in medical costs down the line!

Socks and Optional Gear

What good are walking shoes when you don't have good socks to go with them? Luckily, socks aren't nearly as difficult to figure out as shoes. If you choose to purchase new socks, keep in mind that you're looking for materials that will keep your feet dry and supported. If you plan on walking or exercising long-term (as I hope you do) I recommend investing in a pair of thick socks made of acrylic, polyester, or a wool blend that will keep your feet from getting too wet while you walk. Wet feet can lead to some nasty fungal infections, athlete's foot, and uncomfortable blisters—and a lot of common materials like cotton can contribute to this.

On the other hand, you also don't want your socks to be too constricting—aim for socks that will keep your feet dry while simultaneously letting your feet breathe. As we talked about at the beginning of the chapter, your surroundings are important as well. Look for a pair of thicker socks to keep your feet warm if it's wintertime, and a pair of thinner breathable socks to keep your feet cool in the summertime. As always, make sure that your socks fit well. If you plan to add daily walking to an already-existing exercise regimen, you might also want to look into compression socks. Compression socks are excellent for runners or people who regularly participate in moderate or high-intensity exercise, as they can improve blood flow and increase oxygen levels. Beginning walkers probably don't need to invest in compression socks, but they are a great option for those who need a recovery boost after intense activity.

Once your feet feel comfortable, it's time to consider the rest of your body. As usual, the clothes you wear will depend heavily on your surroundings. If you're walking in southern California in the summer, chances are that you're going to be wearing very different clothes than someone walking on a chilly Massachusetts morning in winter. With that in mind, it's important to prepare beforehand for your climate.

As a general rule, I find that wearing at least two thin layers is the best approach for most climates you walk around in. Similar to the material of your socks, you want the innermost layer touching your skin to be moisture-wicking. Cotton, despite the fact that you might not notice it at first, will keep bacteria-carrying moisture close to your skin—this increases the amount of body odor you experience. I can say from experience that wearing shirts made of polyester and nylon makes for far less discomfort during and after walks. Additionally, most polyester and nylon clothing is partly made of recycled materials, which might make you feel better about buying a shirt specifically for walking (Bolitho, n.d.). That being said, if you live in a hotter climate, cotton's moisture retention may actually cool you down when you exercise (as long as you don't mind being covered in a little perspiration).

Once you have your first layer settled, it may also be a good idea to invest in a lightweight insulating jacket. Alternatively, something like a windbreaker or a waterproof jacket may be better for those living in particularly wet places. Pants should follow the same rules as shirts for exercise—lightweight, moisture-wicking, and thin. Personally, I love wearing yoga pants for walking! Finally, you'll also want to think about color and visibility in your walking clothes. You don't have to pick a neon yellow jacket, but you should make sure that your clothes are somewhat bright and easily visible. If your clothes don't have bright colors, you can also add some reflective strips to clothing you already have.

Once you have your walking clothes sorted out, you may want to add or subtract a few items depending on the climate. Hats, for instance, are great fashion accessories for walkers, and they'll keep your ears warm. Carrying a water bottle on your walks is always a good idea; and if you're planning on walking for some time, you may also want to bring a few healthy snacks. Depending on your environment, you may also want to prepare yourself with things like bug spray and sunscreen.

Preparing yourself for your walk is a very important aspect of safety, but there's a limit to things you can do before you leave your house. For people who are new to exercise walking, knowing basic pedestrian safety precautions is a must. For walkers of all experience levels, it is crucial to examine your surroundings at all times and to be prepared to deal with a variety of unexpected events.

WALKING SAFETY

First things first, let's discuss your environment. As we've covered, all outdoor environments are different and will ultimately require your own research. That being said, there are a few things that you should be mindful of no matter what environment you're in.

Wild animals and other people notwithstanding, just being out in nature for a prolonged time necessitates some foresight and safety knowledge. For one, food and water are major concerns. Taking nature walks, especially in places without many people around, is somewhat similar to being a wilderness survivalist—you must be responsible for and aware of your own bodily health at all times.

These are just some of the considerations you should be cognizant of:

- Are you drinking enough water?
- Are you keeping your energy up with periodic snack breaks?
- What did you eat and drink before you started walking?
- Where is your nearest source of water?
- How far away is civilization?

I know these may seem a bit extreme when you're only going for your daily walk, but a situation can spiral out of control faster than you realize. About an hour or two before you plan to go walking, make sure to drink a tall glass of water. This will hydrate you without putting you on the spot to find a restroom in the middle of your walk. You should also not consume any caffeinated or alcoholic drinks before you walk, as these will impact your body's ability to retain water. When walking for more than an hour or so, it's a good idea to bring along both a water bottle and an electrolyte-restoring drink of your choice. The same precautions should be taken with food—make sure to eat well (but not overeat) before your walk, and bring a few snacks with you just in case. After your workout, make sure to rehydrate and eat again if needed.

You should also keep track of your route, your location, and your general surroundings. In general, you always want to walk in a well-lit, well-traveled area, preferably with paved walkways if you're a beginner. When you're walking outdoors, it's also important to hear what's going on around you. It might seem like an annoyance at first, but wearing only one earbud will allow you to keep track of what's happening in your surroundings, from wild animals to other pedestrians. You always need to keep track of exactly where you are in order to protect yourself and prevent fatigue, dehydration, heat stroke, hypothermia, and a number of other potentially dangerous situations. Having a physical map or digitally downloaded map with you is a great idea, especially if you think you might lose cell phone reception at some point during your walk.

You should also look at the weather forecast before you leave, and consider what other elements you might encounter along your route. Some questions to ask yourself can be:

- Are there going to be animals out and about at this time of day?
- Depending on your region, are there animals or insects that pose a danger to you?
- What should you do if you find yourself in a dangerous situation with an animal?

Of course, you don't have to trek through the wilderness every day if you don't feel like it. With potentially deadly snakes and other animals, I don't blame you! However, urban environments can be just as dangerous as rural areas, perhaps even more so. Just as with more rural environments, you'll want to stay in well-lit, well-defined areas that preferably have a designated walkway. Wearing only one earbud is even more important in urban areas, considering that you might be able to hear a car before a driver sees you. While many cities in the U.S. aren't walkable, try to walk in areas that have smooth, wide walkways and little car traffic. If you are walking in an area with car traffic, stay away from narrow shoulders, and always walk facing oncoming traffic.

On that note, let's talk about pedestrian signals and busy crossings. I know jaywalking can be seen as rebellious, but if you're interested in minimizing your chances of getting hit by a car, I suggest following pedestrian signals. To make sure that you're safe to cross, make eye contact with approaching drivers and look at *all* of the oncoming lanes. Unfortunately, pedestrian accidents increased drastically in the past few years, in almost every state in the United States (Romero, 2022). While you can't control every driver in your vicinity, you can certainly make sure that you're doing your part to stay aware of your surroundings. If you don't want to risk trying to walk on trafficked roads at all, you can also try out your city's parks or local trailheads to get away from the traffic.

Wherever you decide to walk outside, make sure to always carry some form of identification. It might be worth putting together a written list of things for emergency personnel to know in case you're injured—this list could inform personnel that you are on medication, have a serious health condition, or just want to take extra precautions. Items such as a flashlight, whistle, and other small survival supplies may also help you feel more prepared for whatever terrain you're walking through. While walking itself is a fairly safe way to exercise, you never know what Mother Nature may throw your way.

WARMING UP AND COOLING DOWN

Now that we have safety measures out of the way, let's move on to your pre- and post-workout routines. Aside from what you eat and drink, warming up and cooling down can also have significant impacts on the quality and long-term effects of your exercise. Both warming up and cooling down generally involve low-intensity activities that gradually work your muscles and essentially change what mode your body is in. Think of it this way—if you were to stick your hand in ice cold water for three minutes, then run your fingers under steaming hot water, you'd probably be in significant discomfort or pain. The same is true for the rest of your body. Without warming up or cooling down, your system doesn't get any time to adjust to the new conditions in which it finds itself, which puts excess stress on your body as a whole. Temperature plays a key role in getting your system both in and out of workout mode, and warming up is especially important for getting enough blood flow to your muscles. As a result, your muscles will be less prone to injury when you increase the intensity of your activity. You'll also be able to see better results from your workouts when you ease yourself into exercising, and you'll recover from difficult exercises more quickly. I can say from firsthand experience that cooling down and stretching after a long walk is the key to avoiding soreness the day after!

The key word to remember here is "gradual." A warm-up consisting of jumping right into a run or stretching your muscles the farthest they can go defeats the purpose of what you're trying to do. Instead, warm-ups and cooldowns should focus on activities with a lower intensity than the main exercise you're doing. For walkers, this normally means some form of stretching or yoga.

Warming Up

Gradually easing yourself into your daily walk, while it may seem redundant at first, is actually a great method for maximizing your physical performance. Aside from simply warming up your muscles (including your heart), warming up with stretches and yoga can:

- **Improve your oxygen efficiency**

Remember the VO2 max value that you figured out during your at-home testing? By heating your body up and opening up your capillaries, your blood flow is increased. When this happens, the oxygen in your bloodstream has an easier time going where it's needed. By doing this gradually instead of jumping in all at once, you are effectively making sure that your body is performing at its best when you begin your workout.

- **Make your muscle movements faster**

While it's a bit strange to think about it in these terms, all of the exercises that you do are determined by either muscle contraction or muscle relaxation. Physiologically speaking, increased blood flow improves nerve transmission and muscle metabolism, making your reaction time faster than it is when you're in a resting state. When you think about it this way, it's easy to see how warming up can make your exercise better—with more blood flowing to your muscles, your muscles are able to do their job better, contracting and relaxing immediately when they pick up signals from your brain.

- **Place you in the right headspace**

Just like how rushing into a workout can render your body more prone to injuries, failing to get yourself in the right mental space can weaken the effects of your walk. By actively making a decision to warm up, you're essentially practicing how to focus on your body. This bodily consciousness is a great way to get yourself more in tune with what you're feeling, what your body needs, and how to improve.

As with your daily walking exercise, your warm-up can be dressed up or down depending on your body's needs. Fortunately, because walking is such a low-intensity exercise, your warm-up can be as short as three minutes (although you can certainly make it longer). You can do a variety of simple standing stretches in those three minutes that will prepare your mind and body for walking, including (but not limited to):

- **Ankle circles**

Lifting one leg slightly off the ground, simply draw a circle in the air with your toes. Do this about 10 times or so, and then switch legs. This will stretch your ankle through its full range of motion, increasing blood flow and preventing sprains or rolls during your walk.

- **Hamstring scoops**

For this stretch, place one heel in front of your foot like you're beginning to take a step. Keeping the toes of your front foot off the ground, hang your arms as low as is comfortable. If you can, you can also grab the toes of your front foot for a deeper stretch. You should feel the stretch along the back of your legs and hamstrings. Hold the stretch for about five seconds, then switch to the other leg. Repeat as necessary.

- **Leg swings**

Start by standing comfortably with your legs about shoulder distance apart. Raise one foot slightly off the ground, and begin swinging it back and forth like you're skateboarding in place. Raise your leg as high as you can while still remaining comfortable, and use the ball of your foot on the standing leg to keep yourself grounded and balanced. You want your hips to act like a hinge for the leg that's swinging, and you want to keep your moving leg relaxed like the motion of a Newton's cradle. If you feel yourself starting to lean to one side, make sure to keep your head and shoulders as parallel to the ground as possible. Once you've done this about 10 times, switch to the other leg.

These leg swings will begin to move blood toward your hip flexors, which are the muscles around your hip responsible for forward and backward motions. In addition to repeating a walking motion without the impact of the ground, you're also working on improving your balance and strengthening your core muscles.

- **Figure 8 leg swings**

Similar to normal leg swings, figure 8 leg swings begin in a relaxed standing position, with one leg raised slightly off the ground. However, instead of simply swinging the leg from front to back, trace a figure eight with the sole of your foot. The center of the figure 8 should be directly under your hips, and you should basically draw a circle in front and behind your body. Repeat this about 10 times on both sides. These leg swings will begin to work a muscle in your upper thigh called the tensor fasciae latae which, along with the surrounding muscles, is basically responsible for rotating your knee out and away from your hips.

- **Quad stretch**

If you've ever done sports of any kind, or watched athletes prepare for their activity, you've probably seen what a quad stretch looks like. In short, stand comfortably with your legs about shoulder width apart. Balancing on one leg, bend one knee and kick your foot up behind you. If you can grab your foot, hold the toe of your shoe up as close to your body as you're comfortable with. Ideally, you should be able to hold the heel of your foot against your behind. If you're not comfortable grabbing your foot yet, or if you're having trouble balancing, try placing one hand on a wall while the other hand holds your shoe. As the name implies, this stretch works your quadriceps, which are the muscles on the tops of your thighs.

- **Hug your knees**

Hugging your knees is a great way to stretch out the back of your legs and lower back, and you may find that it's easier to hold than other stretches. While standing, bring one of your knees up to your chest, or as close to your chest as you can manage. Hold this position for at least five seconds, and then repeat with the other leg. You may find the position more comfortable if you first form a cradle with your hands by interlacing your fingers. If this position is easy for you, try extending the amount of time you hold the position.

- **Open the gate**

This is another stretch that focuses on your hips, and this one is particularly good for those who have hip and joint problems. Standing with your legs shoulder width apart, raise one leg up like you're taking a step forward. Instead of stepping forward regularly, however, you want to raise your knee higher and rotate it away from your body, landing the step with your foot pointed off to the side. By doing this, you're effectively opening up your hips in a lateral movement, increasing your hip mobility and walking stability. If you've ever done the butterfly stretch, open the gate is similar to a standing version of the butterfly. Perform this exercise about 10 times on each side.

- **Pelvic loops**

Pelvic loops are somewhat similar to what you'd do if you were hula-hooping. Starting with good posture and your knees relaxed, move your hips in a circular motion. Once you've completed 10-15 rotations in one direction, switch directions and hula-hoop the opposite way. Just like hula-hooping, pelvic loops are great for improving the flexibility of your joints and hips and they activate your quads, hip flexors, hamstrings and calves, and strengthen the muscles in your lower back.

- **Arm circles**

Holding your arms out to either side of you, start with both arms parallel to the ground. Begin to make small circles in the air with your fingertips, gradually increasing the size of the circles as your muscles work. Remember to make the circular motions slowly, so as to properly contract each muscle as you move. Do this for about 20 seconds, and then reverse the direction of the circles.

- **Spinal twists**

If you're familiar with yoga at all, you probably know spinal twists as a sitting exercise. However, you can also do less intense spinal twists while standing upright. To start, put your arms out to either side of you like you're doing arm circles. Keeping your feet planted in place, rotate your torso from one direction to the other, twisting your back muscles. While you might not feel as big of a stretch as you would with sitting spinal twists, you will still ultimately be able to warm up the muscles in your back before you walk.

- **Shoulder rolls**

For this exercise, begin by relaxing your shoulders as completely as you can. Then in a circular motion bring them forward, up toward your ears, back, and then down. For a bigger stretch, see how far you can stretch your shoulders down while maintaining proper posture. Roll your shoulders in one direction about 10-15 times, then reverse the direction of the circle.

- **Hula-hoop jumps**

If you're going on a longer walk, hula-hoop jumps are an excellent way to hype yourself up. To begin, start hopping in place. The hops don't have to be big, but you should be jumping at least three or so inches off the ground. As always, remember to maintain good posture by keeping your back straight, and face and shoulders forward. Imagine you're jumping on a clockface—before you initiate the hula-hoop aspect, your feet should be pointing at 12 o'clock each time you land. Next, begin twisting your lower body like you would with a spinal twist. Each time you hop, your feet should be facing at either 9 o'clock or 3 o'clock. At first, you may want to go a bit slower until you get the hang of it. In total, you should jump about 20 times.

With these stretches and movements as a base, you have a great selection of warm-ups to choose from. You don't have to do all of them if you don't want to (you only need about three minutes of warm-up, after all), and you can also spice up your warm-ups by searching for additional exercises. After you feel warmed up, it's time to hit the pavement!

Cooling Down

Despite what you might be thinking, a cooldown session at the end of your walking workout is crucial for long-term results. Again, you don't want to shock your body by abruptly stopping all movement. Additionally, the longer you cool down, the better your chances are of avoiding soreness, tightness, and further injury. As said by Houston-based Dr. Corbin Hedt, "Muscle soreness occurs because muscle and the connective tissue around it get damaged during exercise" (McCallum, 2021). Don't worry, though—this damage that happens during exercise is actually what you want to happen. Often occurring in the form of micro tears, this damage allows your muscles to grow and get stronger. Unfortunately, the cause of soreness is unavoidable, but you can help your muscles recover quicker by using them at a lower intensity than in your workout. For daily walkers, the best way to accomplish this is through static stretches, which are stretches that you simply hold and then release. As with warm-ups, cooldowns should be at least three minutes long (or even longer if you'd like to minimize soreness as much as possible).

Some excellent cooldown options include stretches like:

- **Hamstring stretching**

First things first, you might want to find a yoga mat or a comfortable rug to sit down on. Sitting with one leg fully extended, tuck your other leg in like you would when you're sitting in the tailor sitting position (criss cross applesauce). Next, reach your fingertips toward the toes on your extended leg, and stretch as far as you're comfortable. If you can reach your toes, great! Grab onto your toes, hold the position for about 30 seconds to 1 minute, then switch to the other leg.

- **Calf stretching**

For this stretch, you'll want to stand arm's length away from a wall. From a standing position, step back with one of your feet like you're doing a mini lunge. Keeping both feet flat on the floor, lean your torso forward and place your hands on the wall for balance. Once you feel the stretch in your calf, hold the position for about a minute and then switch to the other leg.

- **Arm stretching**

This stretch is a classic, and for good reason. Start by holding one arm, fully extended, across your chest at shoulder height. Bend the elbow of your opposite arm to hook underneath the first arm and pull upward lightly, positioning your arms at a 90-degree angle. While doing this stretch, imagine that there are invisible strings around your wrists, pulling each arm upward and outward. Hold this stretch for 30 to 60 seconds, and repeat a couple of times on both sides.

These are great stretches for walkers and athletes of all levels, and it's a great idea to do at least one of the above every time you come back from a walk. If you want to make your cooldown more intense, or if you feel like stretching yourself even further, you might try some basic yoga poses like downward dog or the head-to-knee forward bend. You might want to have a yoga mat to do these stretches, but a mat isn't strictly necessary.

- **Downward dog**

For this stretch, begin in a relaxed standing posture, with your feet shoulder width apart. From here, slowly bend your upper half forward, keeping your feet planted. Sometimes, it helps to imagine that you're rolling forward, one vertebra at a time. Once you're within arm's distance, place your hands on the floor in front of you, creating an upside-down V with your body. During this stretch, keep your back as straight as possible, even if it lifts the heels of your feet off of the ground. It may help you to focus on your lower back and behind, creating a very sharp point on your V-shape. Hold this pose for as long as you'd like, although about a minute should be enough.

- **Head-to-knee forward bend**

This exercise is performed sitting down on the ground. Similar to the hamstring stretch that we just covered, you're going to want to extend one leg in front of you while tucking the opposite foot into your thigh. Unlike the hamstring stretch, however, this forward bend goes farther. The goal is to bend the entirety of your back (including your head) so that your face is directly above your knee. Once you're staring at your knee, grab the ball of your foot and hold for about a minute. Repeat on the other side as necessary.

For older walkers, the lower back may tend to be a focal point for your stretches. To maintain flexibility and mobility in this area, you may want to try some low-intensity stretches like:

- **Standing forward bend**

Starting from a relaxed standing position with your knees relaxed, gently bend forward. Like the downward dog, it's best to do this slowly, rolling forward vertebrae by vertebrae. You also want to make sure that your torso and upper body are completely relaxed, letting your head and neck fall naturally toward your feet. Once you're low enough, try to put the palms of your hands on the floor in front of your feet. If this doesn't work for you, you can also try crossing your arms and holding your elbows behind your knees, or even just extending your arms and holding your hands together behind your back. You can do this pose for as long as you'd like, or for at least 30 seconds or so.

- **Shoulder stretch**

For this stretch, place one hand over your shoulder, as low down on your back as you can reach. Place the other hand under your shoulder, as far up on your back as you can reach. Imagine that your hands are magnets, drawing themselves together halfway up your spine. If your hands can touch behind your back in this pose, try clasping them together for a bigger stretch. Hold this position for about a minute, and then switch both arm positions.

- **Legs up the wall**

This stretch is performed exactly how it is written. Sitting with the right side of your body as close as you can get it to the wall, you're essentially going to turn yourself 90 degrees. From sitting with your side against the wall, lay your back down on the floor and swing your legs up against the wall, making a right angle between the floor and the wall. You can put your arms anywhere you'd like, and after that... relax! This is a great cooldown position if you want to finish the last few minutes of your podcast or audiobook. You can hold this position for however short you'd like, but you shouldn't hold it any longer than about five minutes.

- **Savasana**

Contrary to popular belief among non-yogis, this pose is not just sleeping! The simple premise is this—lie directly on the floor with your arms and legs extended, palms facing up, and feet about hip length apart. From here, simply relax. If you've tried savasana before (without falling asleep), you know that relaxing your body completely can actually be quite tricky. A great trick to try out if you're having trouble is to very slowly clench several individual muscles in your body, then unclench them, releasing all of the energy that might be lingering. Personally, I like to start at the bottom with my toes, becoming aware of all of my toes, and then my ankles, my knees, and so forth. Visualizing this process in your mind's eye tends to help—and you should be taking slow, measured breaths during the entirety of the pose. You can hold this pose for as long as you'd like, and I find that it's a great exercise to do after I finish my workday.

At this point, you're an expert on all the preparation for your daily walks—from pedestrian safety to walking essentials and gear, pre-workout warm-ups, and post-workout cooldowns. Now, you can start your walking routine with complete knowledge of how to care for your body and well-being... right? Walking, while indeed one of the first things we all learn to do in life, can actually become surprisingly complicated the more you think about body mechanics. Most of us walk at least a few steps every day, but long-term and long-distance walking requires you to think more actively about what your body is doing. In the next chapter, we'll go over the mechanics of walking, as well as some methods that you can use to make your walking workout as effective and efficient as possible.

4

WALKING TECHNIQUE AND SETTING YOUR OWN PACE

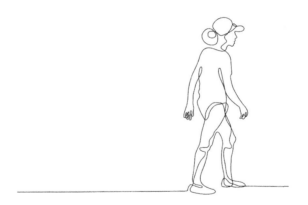

> *An early-morning walk is a blessing for the whole day.*
>
> — HENRY DAVID THOREAU

Every so often, I'll become acutely aware of my walking technique. I begin to overthink very little motion, wondering whether or not I'm moving correctly. Eventually, the feeling subsides, and I continue on my walk normally. During these periods, I always end up questioning my gait, my posture, and even the tilt of my head. It was only when I became interested in the physiology and body mechanics of walking that I realized the importance of all these things. While slightly uncomfortable to think deeply about, it turns out that I was right to analyze my movements. Walking is arguably a big part of what separates humans from other animals, so it's easy to disregard bodily awareness and just put one foot in front of the other. However, the way in which you walk can actually determine the health outcomes you experience.

BENEFITS OF PROPER POSTURE AND GOOD WALKING TECHNIQUE

While there isn't strictly a *correct* way to walk, there are certainly several incorrect (and harmful) ways of walking. In some instances, walking incorrectly can actually result in poor health outcomes such as injuries, joint issues, and other painful conditions. Compared to walking with poor posture, those who walk correctly will see results like:

- **Increased energy levels**

When you're not standing or walking with the right posture, your bones, joints, and cardiovascular system are all affected. Because your bloodstream and your muscles have to work harder to do what they need to do, you'll notice that you use up more energy when you are slouched or too tense. These two factors can in turn impact a variety of things like nutrient uptake, circulation, and metabolism—as well as making you feel sore and stiff. On the other hand, when you walk with good posture, you're essentially making your body more efficient at its job and maximizing the energy you have.

- **Improved lung function, respiratory health, and VO2 max outcomes**

According to the Vancouver Island Health Authority, "If you are tense, your muscles use more oxygen, so keep your shoulders and chest relaxed," while you walk ("Walking and Breathing," n.d.). If your body is out of alignment, it can't function the way it's supposed to. This is perhaps most noticeable through your breathing and heart rate, which can be a big indicator of whether or not you're walking with a relaxed posture. Those who consistently carry good posture will be able to use their oxygen more efficiently and improve their target heart rate while exercising.

- **Improved circulation and heart health**

While most of us have been told to sit with proper posture, how many of us actually do it? If you're slouched or sitting all day at a desk job, chances are that you're carrying over poor posture into your walking exercise. This poor posture can cause blood to pool in the feet and legs, which can cause numbness or discomfort. Additionally, if you're relatively sedentary, your circulation is already suffering simply from sitting for prolonged periods. Meanwhile, those who walk every day with good posture will be able to counter effects like numbness or tingling due to poor circulation.

- **Better digestion**

Walking with poor posture is bad enough, but walking with poor posture after you've just eaten can actually be worse. While walking is a great way to help your body digest food, you also need to make sure that you're not slouching or rolling your shoulders too far forward while you're moving. In the words of Massachusetts General Hospital gastroenterologist Dr. Kyle Staller, "'Slouching puts pressure on the abdomen, which can force stomach acid in the wrong direction,' and, 'some evidence suggests that transit in the intestines slows down when you slouch'" (3 Surprising Risks," 2021). Otherwise, you might end up with some uncomfortable side effects like acid reflux and heartburn. How could one avoid this? By maintaining good posture, of course!

- **Increased stability and a stronger core**

At its most basic, good posture is essentially the best way to maintain stability. If your gait is too long or you're leaning too far forward, you're more likely to be physically unstable as you walk. Meanwhile, walking with your body in alignment actually engages your core muscles properly, rather than having other parts of your body try to compensate for your lack of stability.

- **Quicker muscle movements and higher walking speeds**

By now, I'm sure you can see how all of these factors build on one another. When you walk with good posture, you're increasing your circulation, oxygen efficiency, energy efficiency, and balance. In short, all of these factors will help you reach your walking destination faster than their opposites. Walking with bad posture (and by extension poor circulation, poor oxygen uptake, low energy, and poor balance) puts you at risk for achy muscles and reduced health outcomes after your workout.

- **Properly aligned joints and bones, decreasing your chances of injury**

By maintaining your body's natural stability through posture, you're effectively using your body in the way that it was meant to be used—good job! As a result, your body will reward you by protecting you from rolled ankles and sore joints.

- **Reduction in muscle aches and tiredness**

When your muscles are energy-efficient and they have a good amount of oxygen flowing through them, they tend to wear out far less than they would otherwise. Remember those micro tears that we talked about a while back? These harbingers of next-day soreness can be fought off with plenty of blood flow and correct movement—coincidentally, two things that good posture facilitates.

I'll concede—my parents were right when they told me to stop slouching. If your goal is to improve your general health and well-being, walking with proper posture is the way to do it. So, how does one walk properly? Well, if you're like me, it may help to first learn what *not* to do.

Common Walking Mistakes

Walking is a pretty basic skill, but there are actually numerous ways to do it incorrectly. Your body is a complicated piece of machinery, and without being fully aware of your movements constantly, you're more likely to fall prey to one or more of these mistakes:

- **Overstriding**

When I'm struck with that sudden awful awareness of incorrect posture while walking, this is usually the first thing I notice. Overstriding (taking longer strides than you should) is uncomfortable for a number of reasons —namely leaning too far forward and making your steps louder than normal. Usually, people overstride when they're walking because they're trying to go faster. When you examine what's happening to your body, however, overstriding actually makes you expend more energy. By overstriding, you essentially bite off more than you can chew. As a result, when you step too far forward, your weight is distributed across a wider space, making it land harder. This hard step landing can also have physical effects (in addition to making your steps louder, less efficient, and more uncomfortable). If you overstride consistently, you may experience compression in your joints, knees, and the heels of your feet.

- **Wearing the wrong shoes**

By now, I'm sure you're aware of the importance of good walking shoes. In the previous chapter, we discussed a few factors such as arch support, heel height, and sizing. When you're wearing the right shoe for your foot, you should feel very comfortable while walking. When you're wearing the wrong shoe, however, you will immediately notice the side effects. Aside from being uncomfortable, sore, and achy in the short term, you're also putting yourself at risk for weak joints, injuries, and long-lasting discomfort.

- **Walking flat-footed**

In the same way that wearing the wrong shoes is bad for your joints, walking with flat feet can also have terrible effects. Normal raised arches are basically built to evenly distribute your body weight across the sole of your foot, keeping the weight off of the inside of your legs. When this doesn't happen (or when your arches fall) the majority of your body weight falls where it shouldn't—along the inside of your legs. This can lead to muscle strain, an unstable gait, leg and back pain, and musculoskeletal issues. Paradoxically, flat feet can also negatively affect your posture, compounding the issue and making symptoms of poor posture more noticeable.

- **Too much arm movement or too little arm movement**

When you're walking, arms seem like a strange thing to focus on, considering that they're not immediately essential to the motion of stepping forward. However, walking is a full-body exercise. Your arms can play a big role in the health outcomes you see, and walking without considering your upper body will become obvious if you're doing it incorrectly. Too much arm movement, in addition to looking a bit silly, can impact your balance and gait as you move, priming you for soreness and discomfort. Alternatively, too little arm movement can impact your speed, as well as lead to some uncomfortable swelling in your palms, wrists, and fingers.

- **Head posture**

Unfortunately, many of us are prone to poor head posture when we're walking—myself included. It's easy to change from a good walking posture to a poor one when you pull out your phone to change the music. The same thing can happen when you're reaching around in your pockets, looking down at your feet, or looking down at your dog. For the record, bad head posture is completely understandable—looking down is sometimes necessary so you don't trip over cracked concrete or step on a doggie bag. If you shouldn't look down while you're walking, then where should you look? In general, you should normally be looking slightly ahead of you, about 10 to 20 feet. This will allow you to stay aware of your surroundings, while still being able to see things on the ground that you're approaching. A good rule of thumb is to try to keep your chin parallel to the ground.

- **Leaning**

Leaning can happen for a variety of reasons, but you can generally fix leaning with strength training in your core and back muscles. If you are leaning too far forward or backward while walking, this may indicate that your muscles need some extra attention.

Unintentionally leaning can lead to soreness, muscle weakness, poor circulation, and less efficient breathing. In addition to beginning minor strength training exercises for your back and core, a more immediate fix comes in the form of proper posture—keeping your head up, standing up straight, and relaxing your shoulders.

What Does a Good Walking Technique Look Like?

First things first, good posture starts with body awareness. Additionally, by knowing about common walking and posture mistakes, you're even more equipped to start walking more efficiently and comfortably. Once you're aware of what *not* to do, you can start thinking more critically with each step. It may be overwhelming to take in at first, but it will improve your posture to start walking. A good walking technique includes:

- **Proper heel-to-toe movement**

While runners usually stride from the middle of the foot to the toe, pushing hard off of the ground, walkers should endeavor to make more of a circular motion with their steps. With each stride, you should essentially be working your foot through its full range of motion—from your heel, to the ball of your foot, to your toes. When you land on your heel, make sure to land in the center of your heel, as landing on the very edge of your heel will probably make you lose balance. From here, simply roll your foot from back to front, pushing off the ground with your big toe. As you go through the motion of stepping, increase the amount of force your back foot is exerting on the ground.

Sounds simple enough, right? However, many people don't walk exactly like this. To help you see how you stride, try sitting on a chair with your legs fully extended out in front of you. Then, point the toes of one foot up toward the ceiling with your heel pushed out, and point the toes of the other foot forward like you're trying to touch something in front of you. Then, switch positions from one foot to the other, rolling from heel to toe slowly. If you notice that some muscles in your legs are getting worn out quickly, this probably means that you need to strengthen these muscles to walk properly from heel to toe.

- **Using the proper stride**

Your stride (how long of a distance there is between your steps) depends on a variety of factors like height, weight, and gender. As we mentioned earlier, over-striding can present a big problem for your joints over time. The best way to avoid this is to simply start walking at a comfortable, moderate pace. You don't have to measure your stride down to the inch, but you should generally pay attention to the length of your strides. If you're taking short strides and it feels uncomfortable, lengthen your strides, and vice versa. Your strides may also naturally change if you walk properly from heel to toe, and this is perfectly fine. If you plan to measure distances you walk through the number of steps you achieve (as with most built-in fitness trackers on smartphones), you might want to have a more exact idea of your stride length. However, you can also simply plan out your route through a map or GPS to see how far you've walked.

- **Keeping your body in a straight line**

When you think of posture, your mind probably goes to physical alignment first. Keeping your body in a straight line is a basic but effective way to think about posture, and visualizing this straight line can help while you're actively moving. To do this, imagine that your toes, knees, hips, shoulders, and head all follow a straight line. You essentially want to keep all of these parts within the line, without swaying or leaning left to right or forward to backward. Keeping your feet and eyes forward tends to help with this. Your core muscles should be engaged while you're moving around in order to keep your center of balance, and you should aim to be as tall as you can while still remaining comfortable.

- **Using appropriate arm movements**

Arm and hand position can be tricky to figure out at first, so it's best to keep your elbows bent and keep your arms pumping at a comfortable speed. In general, it helps to think about the relationship between the speed of your arms and legs—your arms can only pump as fast as your legs can walk, so make sure that all of your limbs are in sync with each other. Think about those power walkers whom you might have seen in your neighborhood, the ones who vigorously move their arms as they walk. While this might feel silly at first, you may benefit from trying to imitate them in order to get your bearings. That being said, try not to move your arms too much or raise them above the level of your chest. Additionally, you want to make sure that your hands are relaxed, but not limp.

With all of these aspects in mind, you're all set to hit your favorite trail or walkway! It might take some adjustment at first, but good posture will ultimately set you up for good health outcomes. Over time, these adjustments will become second nature, and you'll be able to reap the benefits of all of your hard work and effort.

CREATING SUSTAINABILITY

Now that we have all of your immediate walking needs met, let's take a second to examine some long-term practices to keep your routine working well. Remember: One of your main goals in adopting a new health routine is to make it stick. Sustainability is what separates a healthy lifestyle from a temporary social media health fad. One key to this is accessibility, which you might have already accomplished by integrating walking into your daily life. Another key to this is to take care of your broader health outside of walking. A great way to keep your walking sustainable is to allow yourself room to rest and recover between workouts. Make sure to not overtrain as well—passion for your new health regimen is amazing, but you don't want to burn yourself out. A sustainable routine may include integrating different exercises of different intensities into your day. You don't have to walk for an hour every day, and it might actually benefit you to shorten your walks on days when you're doing strength or flexibility training.

Additionally, it will help you in the long run if you know what skill level you fall into. If you've already been walking consistently for several years, chances are that the ways in which you need to keep your routine sustainable differ from someone else's who has just started walking. By knowing your skill level, you'll be able to determine approximately where you should be, as well as what type of general schedule and metrics you need to adhere to during your workouts. No matter what skill level you're at, you should feel challenged but not exhausted. Your long-term routines may take some adjusting to find your perfect fit:

- **Beginners** should feel relatively comfortable walking about 10 minutes per day, at around a pace of 3 miles per hour. For context, this means that a beginner would comfortably walk a mile in about 20 minutes or so. A good routine for beginners might include slowly increasing the amount of time you walk—starting at 10 minutes per day and growing to 30 minutes per day (consistently more every day!).
- **Intermediate walkers** are usually in pretty good shape before they start adopting their new routines, so they're able to start at a slightly more rigorous level. Intermediate walkers generally walk somewhere between 3.5 to 4.5 miles per hour, resulting in a mile being

covered between 13-17 minutes. Intermediates should aim to complete about 2 to 3 miles on every walk.
- **Advanced walkers** are already comfortable covering longer distances at relatively higher speeds. These types of walkers may include former athletes or those who live an already active lifestyle. For these people, additions like weights, inclines, sandy beaches, and racewalking are all great choices to make sure you're challenged enough in your daily routine.

Setting Realistic Goals

The goals you set when you first start walking may often fall short of what your body actually needs. You may need to increase or decrease the level of challenge you're giving yourself, and you may find that some workouts are outliers. All of this is normal, and there's no shame in adjusting your goals to better fit your needs and your skill level. In fact, routinely analyzing your goals and your current situation is simply part of living a sustainable and healthy lifestyle, as you're always growing and changing. No matter what your skill level is, you should try to aim for the daily minimum of 30 minutes of moderate- to low-intensity exercise recommended by the Surgeon General

("Exercise: Starting," n.d.). That said, undershooting the recommendations for one or two days per week isn't going to destroy your physical health. As long as you're making a true, concerted effort to improve your health, you're bound to see results.

With this baseline of 30 minutes per day for most days throughout the week, you'll hopefully be able to eventually start setting goals of your own. If you're walking to achieve weight loss, for instance, now is the time to start thinking about what metrics you want to hit. You can ask yourself the following questions:

- Do you want to lose 20 pounds?
- How long do you want to keep the weight off?
- How many calories do you want to burn?
- Is there a specific number you're aiming for?

The more detailed you can be about your goals, the better of an understanding you'll have of how to get there. The same can be said for all health goals, from kicking a food craving to gaining muscle and becoming stronger. Depending on your own goals, body, skill level, and situation, you'll be able to start determining your own walking schedule and intensity intuitively. For those seeking weight loss, this might look like a daily walking workout that hits your target heart rate (moderate intensity) combined with calorie reduction, portion control, and dietary improvements.

For those looking for a general-purpose routine to stick to, there are several resources online that can give you a good idea of what to aim for. For instance, the U.S. National Heart, Lung, and Blood Institute has a 12-week long routine for beginners, which can serve as a great basis for your long-term routine (Mayo Clinic Staff, 2021a). The routine looks like this:

Week	Warm-up	Walk	Cooldown
1	5 minutes	5 minutes	5 minutes
2	5 minutes	7 minutes	5 minutes
3	5 minutes	9 minutes	5 minutes
4	5 minutes	11 minutes	5 minutes
5	5 minutes	13 minutes	5 minutes
6	5 minutes	15 minutes	5 minutes
7	5 minutes	18 minutes	5 minutes
8	5 minutes	20 minutes	5 minutes
9	5 minutes	23 minutes	5 minutes
10	5 minutes	26 minutes	5 minutes
11	5 minutes	28 minutes	5 minutes
12	5 minutes	30 minutes	5 minutes

As you can see, the entire workouts are pretty minimal —workouts for your first week are only 5 minutes, making the entire process just 15 minutes long. Even at the program's height, you're still only working out for less than an hour. If there's an hour-long podcast episode that you've been meaning to listen to, now's the time to queue it up!

Of course, your starting point will ultimately depend on your body. Every situation is unique, and you may require some additional footholds from which to jump into your new walking routine. Aside from doing your own research, it's wise to schedule a visit with your general practitioner to make sure that a schedule like the one above is a good choice. In particular, you should definitely seek professional guidance if you:

- have been sedentary for a year or more
- don't exercise consistently and are over the age of 65
- have been diagnosed with a cardiovascular condition
- are currently pregnant
- have consistently high blood pressure (hypertension)
- have type 2 diabetes
- experience chest pain when you exert yourself
- often feel faint or experience severe dizzy spells or vertigo
- have been diagnosed with other medical conditions that prevent you from walking easily

Many of the above conditions will greatly impact how you walk and exercise, and walking may intensify the symptoms you experience. Additionally, symptoms like frequent vertigo, fainting spells, and chest pain upon exertion are potentially indicative of an underlying medical condition. If you experience any of these (that haven't yet been attributed to a medical condition), the chances of injury are potentially riskier because you don't have medications or practices to alleviate the symptoms. The only person who really knows your body is you, but professional medical advice can give you essential information about how to best care for your health. If you choose this 12-week plan after receiving a go-ahead from your doctor, it may benefit you to also begin incorporating strength training into your routine. Push-ups, planks, and squats are all great exercises for those looking to improve heart health and strength, and repetitive strength exercises are great for people who are trying to lose weight.

Hopefully by now, you have a basic grasp of proper walking posture, how to create an environment of sustainability for your physical health, and the conceptualization of workout scheduling. In the next chapter, we'll dive into some tips for where to walk outdoors, how to optimize your walking experience, and some advice for nature-lovers.

ENJOYING THE GREAT OUTDOORS

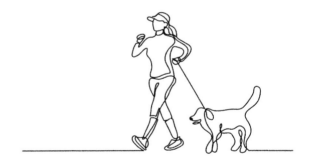

A walk in nature walks the soul back home.

— MARY DAVIS

Despite growing up in a big city, I adore being outdoors. There's nothing that beats a warm, sunny day and a long hike through dense trees. For me, walking out in natural landscapes presents an opportunity for me to reconnect with my senses. *What am I hearing? What am I smelling? Are the leaves changing color?* Almost every time I walk outdoors, there's something new that surprises me. Being the only person around to see a falcon fly overhead, or watching a river turtle munch on some foliage is somehow deeply humanizing. I am part of a natural system, and being able to take part in it is comforting. There's something about walking outdoors that reinforces my mental health, and I always return feeling strong, rejuvenated, and connected with the world around me.

Of course, not everyone enjoys the outdoors. With bugs, animals, and a whole world of potentially harmful plants and organisms, I understand where the hesitation comes from. However, before you decide to shut your front door and stay indoors, I would urge you to listen to the science behind heading outdoors. You might find that, despite the chance of mosquito bites, there are more rewards than consequences.

WHY WALK OUTDOORS?

Many of the initial physical benefits of walking outdoors that one might point to (like lowering your blood pressure, staving off extra weight, and kick-starting basic cognitive function) don't necessarily need to happen outside. If you'd like, you can technically omit the term "outdoor" and still reap some amazing physical benefits. However, your brain is a complicated machine. Over the course of thousands of years, the human brain has developed some very strong connections with nature—both physiologically and psychologically. While we don't quite know how it all works yet, there is ample evidence suggesting that exercising outdoors (preferably in local natural surroundings) is the best way to get your walking workout in and simultaneously improve your mental health.

In one 2020 analysis of studies published by the American Psychological Association, science writer Kirsten Weir explains that walking outdoors, specifically in nature, "has been linked to a host of benefits, including improved attention, lower stress, better mood, reduced risk of psychiatric disorders, and even upticks in empathy and cooperation" (Weir, 2020). Here is our problem—how do we separate the basic effects of walking from the more specific effects of walking in nature? Luckily, many, many scientists have been asking the same thing.

At the University of Washington in 2019, Dr. Gregory Bratman shared an analysis of years of studies in research, and found a recurring theme—walking through nature is empirically linked to a better emotional state, improved social interactions between people, higher reported rates of happiness, and lower rates of mental disorders. The trends from the meta-analysis didn't stop there, either. Data from several studies suggested that interacting with nature and looking at natural scenes even gave people a heightened sense of purpose (Bratman et al., 2019). Mind you, this isn't one study conducted in one place during a limited time frame. The analysis included research from all over the world including various age groups, ethnicities, and backgrounds.

Additionally, further studies have suggested that these effects are lasting. In another 2019 study, this one out of Denmark, scientists found that children who were raised around a natural setting saw massive declines in psychiatric and psychological disorders. On the other hand, children who grew up without any access to nature or green space were prone to mental illnesses at a 55% higher rate (Weir, 2020). In short, out of a whopping 900,000 participant pool, those who interacted with nature regularly (or even just saw nature in their day-to-day lives) saw dramatically improved health outcomes.

With that in mind, a couple of mosquito bites do not seem so bad.

There is also ample evidence to suggest that exercising outside is better for you physically. According to one Massachusetts-based neurotherapy clinic, air quality may play a factor in the physical effects you see (Advanced Neurotherapy PC, 2020). While air quality is highly dependent on your location, it's easy to see how sitting in stale air inside an office could translate into lower blood oxygen levels. The same could be argued for your home, where air tends to sit unless you have windows open and fans on.

Walking outdoors, on the other hand, can provide your brain and muscles with some much-needed fresh air. Similarly, the ground you walk on at home or in other indoor settings can make a difference in your workout. Outdoors and in nature, where the ground varies in hardness and terrain, you are essentially forced to pay attention and adapt to your surroundings. While building awareness of your body more generally, health experts like NCAA distance coach Sean Fortune also believe that inconsistent ground builds more strength than flat indoor ground like that of a treadmill. In one

GQ interview, Fortune states, "You don't build the same strength in the musculoskeletal system, since the treadmill platform is relatively soft'" (Schultz, 2018).

Additionally, there is one thing outdoors that your office space or home will never be able to replicate: Sunlight! Vitamin D is a crucial nutrient that your body needs to keep your immune system up and running. Unfortunately, for a wide population of people in 136 countries around the world, vitamin D deficiency is a big problem (Haq et al., 2016). In the United States, an estimated 40% of people have a vitamin D deficiency, which is made more difficult to overcome by the fact that vitamin D is not found in many foods commonly eaten in America (Raman, 2018). As a result, this part of the population is more prone to conditions like osteoporosis, cancer, depression, and muscle weakness—all of which we've already discussed in correlation with a sedentary lifestyle. Depending on your geographical location, this is easily remedied by spending just 10 to 30 minutes outdoors when the sun is shining (Raman, 2018).

OUTDOOR WALKING EXERCISES

Outdoor walking, by virtue of being environmentally inconsistent, is already a great way to engage your body and mind. If you're not totally convinced yet, you should know that there are also different types of outdoor walking you can do. You might wonder how there can be different types of walking when the activity itself is so simple.

Part of the beauty of walking is its variability. Spicing up the scenery, method, or engagement process involved in your daily workout is a great way to build strength and body awareness. In addition, everyone's situation is different. If you can't carve out an hour's worth of walking every day, then your walking routine will look very different from someone who is retired and has plenty of time on their hands. Fortunately, the simple act of walking is almost universal—you can walk almost anywhere, at any time, with (or without) anyone. To give you an idea of what I'm talking about, let's examine some of your outdoor options:

- **Urban commuting**

For those of us with that pesky office job or in-person nine-to-five, here's your walking solution. Urban commuting essentially describes walking with an urban purpose—like taking the bus, heading to work, or grabbing lunch at your favorite spot. Usually, urban commuting is most compatible with—you guessed it—people inhabiting urban areas. If you live in a walkable area of the suburbs, with proper walkways and safe pedestrian areas, you might be able to squeeze a couple of miles into your day.

- **Afghan walking**

Named after the place where it was first developed, Afghan walking is a method of walking which lines up your breathing patterns with your strides. While it sounds simple in theory, Afghan walking is a great way to practice proper posture, good breathing, and body awareness. Afghan walking requires you to breathe through your nose at all times, and usually goes something like this: Take three steps forward, inhaling through your nose for the entirety of those steps, and then exhale through your nose on the fourth step. This pattern usually increases incrementally, gradually building up the number of steps you take with each inhale.

- **Marathon walking**

Marathon walking (sometimes also called sport walking) is a great option for those who want to build up their endurance. Just like a regular running marathon, these marathon walking events usually take you through different parts of an urban area for a total distance of about 26 miles. While still maintaining a moderate to high intensity, marathon walking gives you the chance to enjoy the scenery while still getting your endurance workout in.

- **Nordic walking**

Perfect for people who love skiing but hate the snow, Nordic walking requires that you bring two walking poles on your walk with you. While walking normally, practitioners use the poles to push off of the ground behind them, effectively strengthening and stabilizing their back legs as they walk. While you should be careful not to harm the trails or nature you're walking on, Nordic walking can present a perfect opportunity to engage your arms while moving your lower body.

Taking Your Workouts to the Next Level

Personally, when I hear the term "workout," pleasure isn't the first thing that springs to mind. Sure, being out in nature can be lovely (and post-exercise endorphins do wonders for my mood and energy), but the physical sensations of working out aren't really my favorite. Walking, in part because it's a very simple activity, is sometimes difficult to focus on because it's so low-intensity. Even when you're out and about in nature, your walking workout may still be a little…unengaging.

If this sounds familiar, you might want to add some more elements to your walking sessions, including:

- **Walking with intention**

Planning a simple routine, like the 12-week routine we covered earlier, is great—but there's always more you can do. Each week, try planning out what your intentions are before you walk. For instance, one day might focus on building leg strength by carrying weights, and another day might focus on endurance by increasing your distance. Whatever your intentions are for your workout sessions, try explicitly spelling them out for yourself in as much detail as you can muster. Writing things down can also help you hold yourself accountable and stick to your plan.

- **Walking routes with elevation**

If you've ever tried to climb a flight of stairs quickly, you know that trying to walk upward is harder than walking on a flatter surface. The same can be said for hills, mountains, or even sandy dunes. In addition to expending more energy (and burning more calories), walking on an incline of some kind will help you work your glutes more than you would on an even surface.

- **Making it a competition**

Sometimes, the best challenges present themselves through metrics. Competing with other people is great, but you can also compete with yourself. How fast you can walk a trail or the distance of a walking route are great metrics to use as starting points. On your next walk, try timing yourself—how long did it take you to walk one mile? Make a note of it, so you can try to beat that time the next time you walk.

- **Trying to push your metrics**

You don't have to time yourself or compete with yourself to grow. Depending on where you are in your fitness journey, consider trying to maximize your workout to the best of your ability. If you walked three miles today, for instance, try your best to up the ante. Even another tenth of a mile can make you feel more accomplished and more refreshed than you otherwise would be. The same thing can be done with the number of steps you do, as well as the time you spend working out.

- **Finding trails you love**

As we mentioned earlier, trails often present a great way to both view nature and strengthen your feet and ankles. However, you may find that you like some trails more than others. As you begin your walking routine, try to explore the trails in your area and see which ones suit you. Do you prefer paved trails, or do you like trails with unpaved walkways? Which trails have the best lighting? Do you want to walk on popular trails, or do you prefer less traffic on your walk? As always, your route is entirely up to you, so here's your chance to make the most of it!

In short, walking outdoors in natural settings is great for your physical and mental well-being. However, not everyone has the access or desire to walk outside. If you're anywhere in America, from big cities to remote rural towns, you already know that walkable areas are somewhat limited. In the next chapter, we'll discuss what to do when you *can't* walk outside, or when walking outside is not an option.

6

WALKING INDOORS

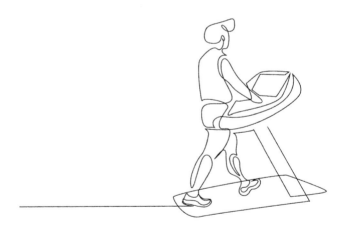

> *Walking: the most ancient exercise and still the best modern exercise.*
>
> — CAROL BECK

For many Americans, walking outside can be unenjoyable, but also potentially dangerous. It may be difficult to recognize while you're living a thoroughly modern lifestyle, but our culture and social infrastructure (and even our homes) are sometimes antithetical to physical and mental health. That statement is all well and good to make, but what does this actually look like for the average person? Before we look at why outdoor walking is not the best idea for everyone, let's examine the definition of the term "walkability." In simple terms, walkability describes a community's ability to comfortably navigate around an area on foot. According to the website Walkscore.com ("What Makes," n.d.), which measures walkability across the United States, a walkable community requires at least six different factors:

- a neighborhood center, like a main street or a community park
- locals with mixed income, often indicated by affordable housing near local businesses
- ample parks and public spaces
- good pedestrian designs across the area, like businesses that are close to the street and parking lots that don't interfere with walkways
- schools and workplaces that are close to local businesses and green spaces

- completed streets, with relatively even and accessible sidewalks, bike lanes, and shade

As you can see, these requirements make the pool of walkable cities and towns smaller, in large part due to the prevalence of cars in the United States as the primary means of transportation. This isn't just my opinion—the National Physical Activity Plan coalition (including the American Cancer Society, the American Medical Association, and the American Academy of Pediatrics) conducted a 2017 study of walkability in cities across America. The coalition's findings were dismal at best, with categories like pedestrian infrastructure, safety, institutional policies, public transportation, and youth walking prevalence all scoring a solid "F" (Schmitt, 2017). The "walkable neighborhoods" category scored a "D," which—while better than the lowest score possible—is still a terrifying failure. Most of this stems from a firmly institutional failing, as spending for safe pedestrian infrastructure only comes out to about $2.47 per capita for most states in the country. As a result, people who want to walk outdoors are forced to put their safety in jeopardy. To make matters worse, one study found that the least walkable neighborhoods in the country are usually in low-income or poor areas, with Americans of color receiving even fewer pedestrian opportunities than White Americans (Conderino et al., 2021).

If you live in an area where walking is accessible, many Americans have jobs or careers that prevent consistent hour-long walks. In 2021, the Bureau of Labor Statistics released information about the average American's work week, with most people at work for about 38 hours per week. More specifically, people of both genders from the ages of 25 to 54 worked an average of over 40 hours per week (Doyle, 2022). As you can probably imagine, this issue isn't something that you can budge on—your livelihood and your ability to provide for your loved ones ultimately comes before most other activities. Making the problem of getting outdoors even more insurmountable is the issue of air quality. Even when you live in an area where you feel comfortable walking outside, and even when you have time to walk every day, the air you breathe can still make walking detrimental to your respiratory health. The American Lung Association names big cities like Houston, Los Angeles, and Detroit as having some of the highest rates of particle pollution in the United States ("Most Polluted Cities," 2021).

All of these issues make it difficult for some people to walk outdoors. This doesn't mean that you have to forego walking altogether, however—walking indoors can solve many of the issues that we've outlined. As long as you can find enough space to take a couple of steps, you'll still be able to benefit from the physical and mental impacts of daily walking.

INDOOR WALKING EXERCISES

In many cases, walking indoors can have just as much variety as walking outdoors, especially if you live close to a city center. While you're not getting the benefits of interacting in nature, your indoor exercises don't have to compromise on intensity, speed, or distance. As long as it works for your situation, any step is a good step!

That being said, the way you walk indoors is going to be undeniably different from the way you would walk outdoors. This might include walking styles like:

- **The amble**

This style is great for those who are just starting out with walking as an exercise, or for those who just want to admire their surroundings. When you amble, you are slow and relaxed, taking your time to focus on the world around you (while maintaining good posture, of course). This is a great style to use in places like museums, art galleries, or other indoor installations, and it also provides a great way to chip away at your metrics and goals.

- **Casual stroll**

Faster than an amble but slower than a steady walk, a casual stroll is usually performed when you have a casual goal in mind. For instance, you might casually stroll to a low-key business meeting at work, or to the coffee shop in your building.

- **Steady walking**

The steady walk is essentially the standard for most people, and it's a good way to judge your skill level. Steady walking includes consistent pacing and intensity —not too fast but not too slow. When you're walking steadily, you should be able to have a full-length conversation without getting tired or out of breath.

- **Brisk walking**

Relative to steady walking, brisk walking involves slightly more energy expenditure. In other words, a long conversation during a brisk walk might make you run out of breath a little. Unlike strolling or ambling, brisk walking tends to offer more health benefits as a result of its faster pace.

- **Sport walking**

Sport walking is a bit like brisk walking and Afghan walking combined—a brisk pace is required, in addition to careful breathing and pace. Additionally, sport walking is best suited for flat environments, making it perfect for indoor walkers.

- **Meditative walking**

For those looking for a mental health boost, meditative walking is the best option. While you're not reaping the benefits of being outdoors, mindful or meditative exercising indoors can still improve your mood, concentration, and affect. This type of walking doesn't require any particular pace, environment, or breathing techniques, making it perfect for an indoor setting. There aren't really any hard and fast rules for meditative walking, but there are a few types of meditative walking that you might draw inspiration from.

- **Gratitude walking**

As the term suggests, this requires you to make a list of all the things you're grateful for that day, such as your family, career, or circumstances. Did a stranger smile at you on the bus? Did the barista at your favorite coffee shop remember your order from the last time you were there? Did your coworker offer to take some tasks off your plate at work? Anything you're grateful for—even the smallest things in your day-to-day life—can make you more aware and more mindful.

- **Pump-me-up walking**

As an alternative to gratitude walking, you can try pump-me-up walking, which is designed to make you feel more energized and confident. While playing your favorite songs, think about what you need to hear in the present moment. Do you need to hear how good of a spouse you are? Do you need to hear that your input is valuable? During your walk, you are going to effectively be your own best friend, cheering yourself on as if you were talking to someone else.

- **Power walking**

Power walking is perhaps the closest exercise to running that you can perform—without actually running, of course. Power walking happens at a fast pace, usually as fast as you can manage without running, and falls into the high-intensity category as a result. Power walkers use vigorous arm motions in addition to fast-paced steps in order to achieve a full-body workout. Because the goal is to walk as fast as possible, power walking is best done on a flat, even surface, like those that you'd find indoors.

You could also choose to combine two of these walking styles. As always, walking with good posture is a must, and warming up is still necessary even when you don't leave the building. With all of these options to try, you may be wondering how to work these into your daily schedule while not stepping foot outside. Luckily, there are a variety of indoor space options to test out.

Indoor Walking Opportunities

Ultimately, every step is a good step, no matter where it's taken. Even if you're in a small room or office space, walking in place is a completely valid method for hitting your step goals. Are you walking to meet a coworker on the other side of the building? It counts!

Are you walking to the mini fridge in your office? It counts! In fact, just standing up from your desk every so often and taking a short lap around your cubicle is better than nothing. Your space, no matter how small it might look at first glance, can be turned into a workout room with just a slight adjustment in perspective. If you can stand up in a space, you have enough room to get a few steps in, even if you don't go anywhere.

Of course, more space is almost always better. Walking in place, while it might help in meeting your goals, gets a little boring after a while. Fortunately, there are several indoor places where you can walk:

- indoor shopping centers
- art galleries and museums
- schools and college facilities
- gym tracks
- libraries
- grocery stores

Almost anywhere with commercial significance, or anywhere that you might buy something, can present a good option for walking around. When you're at the grocery store, for instance, make sure you survey all of your options before putting something in your cart. Walking around the edge of the store is a good choice, and taking time before buying food will give you the added benefit of considering your diet.

Treadmills

Aside from public places like libraries and art galleries, there is another option that allows you to work out indoors, and possibly in the comfort of your own home. While not ideal, treadmills can be a good opportunity for walking and workout variation catered to your needs. Treadmills have the potential to offer more intense workouts than other machines like stationary bikes or ellipticals, and soft treadmill belts can be great for those who want more consistency in their daily workouts. Those worried about falling or tripping on outdoor surfaces may be more suited to treadmills, and the softness of the treadmill belt won't cause as much wear and tear on your feet and ankles. The downside to this is that your feet, joints, and muscles won't be as strong—but if strength isn't your top priority, a treadmill might be the best option. Alternatively, if you want to simulate the ground outside, you can always vary your incline and increase the speed settings. You should also know that walking on a treadmill uses slightly different muscles than walking outdoors, and your hamstrings in particular might feel a bit more sore than usual after walking on a treadmill.

While a treadmill takes more investment than walking on the ground outside, it's probably not as expensive as you're thinking. Buying your own treadmill is certainly an option, but you can also find treadmills at gyms, offices, and even some coworking spaces. Memberships at these places cost far less than buying your own brand-new treadmill, and if you work or live in an urban area, something like a gym or a coworking space will probably be very convenient. If you have your heart set on having your own treadmill, it might be comforting to know that there's a treadmill for just about all of your walking needs. For those who work from home, a small under-the-desk treadmill or a walking pad is likely the best machine for you. In general, you can expect brand-new treadmills to range from $200 to upward of $2,000.

Using a treadmill can come with a few perks that you wouldn't find with other types of indoor walking. This is a great way to try to optimize your workout with the tools you have, including:

- **Positioning a mirror in front or to the side of you**

If you're comfortable with the idea and have access to a large mirror, putting a mirror to the side of your treadmill can allow you to observe your form while you walk. Watching your indoor form on your treadmill can be a good supplement for other forms of walking that you do, and taking notes on your posture and gait is a good way to establish a baseline for your normal walking posture.

- **Trying out your treadmill presets**

Sometimes making your own route and choosing how long and how far you'll walk can be somewhat of a challenge. Putting a lot of thought into your routine, while it encourages mindfulness, may get tiring after a while. If you're walking outside or indoors, every turn is a choice on your part. In the spirit of making walking accessible, use your treadmill presets. This will allow you to sit back and walk on days when you don't really feel like making decisions.

- **Using inclines**

As previously mentioned, using inclines is a good method for working your hamstrings and increasing your energy expenditure. Rather than going out to find a set of stairs or looking for your nearest hilly region, your treadmill has a variety of inclines ready to go. On days when you want to up your workout game, simply choose from your treadmill's incline options.

- **Experimenting with intervals in your workout**

Previously, we talked a bit about trying out your own intervals on outdoor walks. Treadmills and walk pads, while not as versatile, are an easy alternative to doing intervals outdoors. While most treadmills have presets that determine the length of your intervals, you can also simply increase and decrease the speed of the belt manually to cater to your own needs.

- **Using a fan**

Ultimately, the goal of using your treadmill is to simulate walking outdoors as closely as you can. While it may sound ridiculous at first, using a stand-up fan can make a big difference in how you feel during your exercise. Good airflow can simulate a cross-breeze, keeping your body cool and allowing sweat to evaporate more easily. You'll also find that walking in a well-vented room is much better than walking in a room that's stuffy or too hot.

- **Mixing in bodyweight exercises**

From weighted vests to ankle weights, weighted exercises will spice up your workout in no time. In general, it's best to use weights that were made for wearing, as something like a backpack can impact your posture and gait. Using weights will strengthen muscles in every area of your body while you walk, and using weights regularly is a good introduction to strength training and stationary weight lifting.

No matter what you do, a treadmill will probably never measure up to an outdoor stroll, and you won't reap the same benefits physically or mentally. With this in mind, your ultimate goal should be to simulate walking outdoors when you're on a treadmill. Using fans to simulate a cross-breeze and using inclines are good starting points, but feel free to get creative. Would it help to watch nature videos while you're walking? Are you an avid bird-watcher who would benefit from listening to native bird calls while you're exercising? Your indoor workout doesn't have to be boring or repetitive—your treadmill workout should work for you, just as much as you work for it!

Tips for Indoor Walkers

Whether you're in a grocery store or your own home, there's always something more that you can do for your health. Changing your perspective on the available space is crucial to optimizing your workouts, and although it may take some imagination sometimes, coming up with new and different ways to approach your walking exercises will become simple with practice. To get you started, think about options such as:

- walking around the outside of the grocery store before doing your shopping, thereby getting more steps in and being intentional about what you put in your cart
- walking to communicate with your coworkers instead of sending emails, if you're working at an in-person office job
- taking the stairs and walking up escalators when possible
- taking each bag inside your home one by one after grocery shopping
- walking indoors while you're talking to someone on the phone

Ultimately, walking is walking, no matter how you choose to do it. As long as you feel good about your workouts, you'll meet your goals before you know it! Over time, however, your physical ability will eventually outpace the original goals you set for yourself at the beginning of your fitness journey. When this happens, there's only one thing to do—move the goalpost. In the next chapter, we'll go over how to go about making your workouts more intense as your physical abilities improve, as well as some ways to keep you on track in the long run.

7

GOING A STEP FURTHER

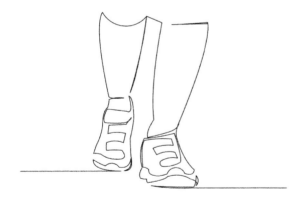

❝ *Life always begins with one step outside of your comfort zone.*

— SHANNON L. ALDER

Think of the last time you mastered something—how did you get there? Practicing the same thing over and over again is all well and good, but simply repeating a skill you already know doesn't do much to further your abilities. Athletes, artists, and creative people of all kinds will know that challenge breeds growth. The only way to improve is to push yourself, and the best growth happens when you push yourself just outside of your current skill level. Otherwise, you will simply remain stagnant. Walking, despite being a low-intensity activity, can in fact be considered a sport. By extension, pushing yourself during your walking exercises is a must if you want to improve posture, strength, and overall physical health. Luckily, because walking is a pretty straightforward activity, there are plenty of ways to further engage your body as you work out.

TAKING YOUR WALKING WORKOUT TO THE NEXT LEVEL

How do you know when you're ready to up the ante on your daily walks? The answer to this question depends on the individual. In general, however, if you can hold a particular pace, distance, or style of walking for one week or more, then you're probably ready for some added challenges. This can be accomplished in a variety of ways, namely through extending distance, increasing your pace, changing your technique, or lengthening the amount of time that you walk. Try challenges such as:

- **The 20-minute speed-it-up walk:** This is performed by 4 minutes of normal walking, followed by 4 minutes of brisk walking. Alternate normal and brisk walking 5 times, for a total of 20 minutes.
- **The 10-minute HIIT walking workout:** This is performed by 4 minutes of normal walking, followed by 2 minutes at an increased pace, 2 minutes at an even faster pace, then 2 minutes of vigorous power walking.
- **The 20-minute walking and strength indoor walking routine:** For this routine, you walk normally around your house for 1 minute, followed by 1 minute of walking in place at a faster pace, and ending with a strength training session including 5 squats, 5 push-ups, and 5 calf raises. Repeat the process until your workout reaches 20 minutes.
- **The upper body walking workout:** While walking normally, alternate 2-minute sessions of forward punches, upward punches, and power-walking-style arm pumping for the length of your walk.

- **The meditative walk:** During your walk, name 5 things you are grateful for about your children, 5 things you are grateful for about your spouse, and 5 things you are grateful for about today's work. If needed, the lists can be altered to better fit your situation.

These challenges can be easily integrated into your daily or weekly routine, and can provide a solid foundation for increasingly difficult challenges. As you're looking to spice up your workouts, you may find that challenges are easier to implement when you're walking with a friend or a pet. For instance, when your dog pulls on its leash, try increasing your pace for five minutes. When your friend suggests exploring a path you have never walked, go see what it looks like. In addition to presenting challenges you may not have thought of yourself, walking with a buddy is also a good method for keeping yourself accountable and motivated.

Tracking Your Results

Of course, baselines and challenges don't really matter when you don't hold yourself accountable for your fitness goals. Personally, one of the main reasons why I've previously struggled with workout regimens is that

I tend to lose track of where I am in my fitness journey. As a result, I end up going in loops and stagnating, eventually falling off the wagon until I decide to try again. To prevent this from happening, there is a stunningly simple solution—keep consistent records.

For starters, making and keeping your physical records requires that you know your metrics. By this, I mean that you need to have a quantitatively *measurable* way of knowing where you currently are. In other words, it's time to bust out the numbers (and maybe your phone's calculator). Qualitative metrics, like a visual inspection of your form, are definitely wonderful to have in your back pocket. Word-based descriptors can eventually allow for some slack into your workouts though, whereas numbers are more definitive. If you have a certain mile time you're aiming for, for instance, there isn't room for a "maybe" in meeting that goal. I find that choosing one or two quantitative aspects to focus on (distance, speed, steps, time, or calories) is the best way to measure yourself. For some, this might look like walking 10,000 steps every day; others might opt for a goal of 30-minute daily workouts. Whatever you choose, make sure to start keeping tabs on yourself as soon as you start. There are several ways in which you could measure your progress, including (but certainly not limited to):

- a physical journal
- a digital log
- a food diary (if you want to focus on caloric metrics)
- fitness trackers and apps such as Argus, Strava, or Runkeeper

After recording your progress for a while, start looking for patterns in your routines. What factors improve the quality of your routine? For me, my physical performance peaks just before midday, when the sun is shining and I'm in between meals. To find out when you're at your best, start looking at things like time of day, weekend versus weekday walks, and solitary versus group walks. Your goal is essentially to find out everything you can about your body, when and where it works best, and how to make it work better. From here, you can start setting more long-term goals for yourself.

That being said, setting goals can be tricky, especially if you're feeling overwhelmed by metrics. Remember to make SMART goals that are:

- **Specific:** stating what needs to happen and how you're going to do it in full detail
- **Measurable:** quantifying your goals through metrics, numbers, and benchmarks

- **Achievable:** reaching just outside of your comfort zone (but not quite shooting for the stars)
- **Relevant:** revolving around your broader health goals, and staying on track
- **Time-based:** when exactly you are going to meet your goals

For example, if you want to start power walking with proper form for five miles per day, and for six days per week, you're more likely to achieve the results you want. If, on the other hand, you simply write "power walk" in your activity journal, you're essentially going to miss all of the details that make your goal feasible. Additionally, you should also work to set both short- and long-term goals, as this will keep you engaged on multiple levels. Short-term goals, like the power walking one above, go hand-in-hand with bigger goals like participating in your city's walking marathon.

Finally, there's one last thing to do: Keep it up! Recording all of your progress, both successes and failures, is the only way to know what's next in your journey. It may seem obvious, but consistently tracking your habits and monitoring your progress is perhaps the most important factor in your improvement over time. Without being able to see how you're doing, you won't know where to improve!

Maintaining a workout journal or database of some kind is a great way to cement your routine into your life. However, you may still experience some mental resistance when you set out on your daily walk. This is perfectly natural, but remember—you want your walking routines to be more than just a phase. As you ease into your routines, you also need to start breaking down some of the mental and behavioral blocks that are stopping you from continuing on your fitness journey. In the next chapter, we'll discuss the mental changes necessary for turning your workouts into lifelong routines through habit building.

8

CREATING YOUR WALKING HABIT

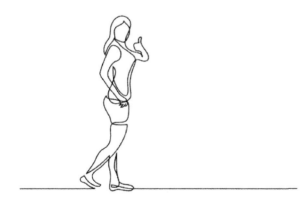

> *A river cuts through rock, not because of its power, but because of its persistence.*
>
> — JAMES N. WATKINS

As cliché as it sounds, your health goals are a marathon, not a sprint. One 10-mile walk doesn't (unfortunately) make up for sitting around for the rest of the week. Like all other acquired skills, your walking abilities improve with small daily segments rather than occasional big bursts of effort. Health and fitness researchers have come to the same conclusion, with one 2022 study finding that those who did smaller workouts 5 times per week reaped bigger results than those who did 30-minute workouts just one time per week. More specifically, the participants who engaged in smaller workouts of 3 to 5 minutes every weekday saw an average 10% increase in strength and a 6% increase in muscle thickness. Meanwhile, the participants who did one big workout just once per week saw no improvements in any area (Dalli, 2022). Furthermore, head researcher Ken Nosaka states, "'Muscle adaptations occur when we are resting; if someone was able to somehow train 24 hours a day, there would actually be no improvement at all'" in their abilities or strength (Dalli, 2022).

At this point, you're hopefully seeing a theme emerge. Those who want to improve in the long term must work consistently, but also give themselves enough time to rest and recover. In this sense, walking and working out every day is very similar to, say, brushing your teeth. Your teeth won't become healthier if you spend four hours brushing them, only to neglect your dental health for the rest of the month. The same can be said for household routines like doing your laundry or watering your houseplants. There's another term for all of these routines—habits.

HOW DO I CREATE HABITS?

The first step in building a sustainable routine is to make your health a habit. What's the difference between a routine and a habit, and why are habits so important in this process? A habit is something you don't even think about—it is a completely automated aspect of your daily life. Habits you probably already engage in include basic hygiene, drinking coffee, and much more. These routines are so incorporated into the fabric of your everyday life that they don't require any extra effort. By extension, habits aren't something that go away easily. Brushing your teeth before bed isn't something that you can simply forget to do. In fact, it sometimes takes more work to undo habits than it does to form them! For people who want to start walking regularly, however, this transition from activity to habit hasn't happened yet. As a result, you may find that it takes some extra effort to get yourself up and moving. Additionally, it may be difficult to figure out exactly *how* to make walking a habit. The key is sticking to the little things, like putting on your shoes after you've had breakfast or charging your Bluetooth headphones before you go to bed. Creating space for your new walking habit through several small adjustments breaks the problem down into bite-sized, easily-tackled pieces.

Let's look at this problem in another way. Essentially, you want to make working out as easy as possible for yourself, while still maintaining the health benefits and structure of the activity. One great way to accomplish this is by considering your physical and mental setting before, during, and after you walk. James Clear, the author of *Atomic Habits*, states that time, location, preceding events, and your emotional state are all crucial in understanding how to put together effective habits (Clear, 2015). Once you understand how to build effective habits, you can begin using these four elements to your advantage:

- **Time**

Starting from the top, time is perhaps the most common way to build habits, in large part because time is easy (and necessary) to measure. For instance, I automatically get up and make coffee at about 7 a.m. in the morning. I know this because after my alarm goes off at 6:30 I stay in bed and read for 30 minutes, then get up and go to the kitchen and look at the clock on my oven. From here, it would be easy to integrate a new habit into the routine because I'm already so aware of the time. Squeezing in a 15-minute walk between the time I get out of bed and the time I make coffee wouldn't be that much of a stretch.

- **Location**

Next, location is also a big factor in building habits. Getting out of your usual setting (namely, your house) is a great start, and assigning different locations for different activities will help you form associations. That one trail that's close to your house might be the perfect place to start implementing your new walking habit, and going there will gradually begin to make you want to walk.

- **Preceding events**

Using preceding events, which are sometimes linked to time, is one of the most effective ways to build habits into routines that already exist. For instance, charging your Bluetooth headphones every time you close your computer for the day is a great way to make sure that you're ready to go on tomorrow's walk. The preceding events in question don't have to be big, mind you—a phone notification, going to bed, or getting up to go get lunch are all great opportunities for you to either walk, or somehow prepare yourself for walking.

- **Emotional state**

Your emotional state is inextricably linked with your body awareness. Oftentimes, your internal feelings bubble up through unavoidable physical responses (like shoulder tension, higher blood pressure, or poor posture), which can all be all fixed with consistent walking. This is when the mind-body connection that we talked about earlier becomes clear, despite the theories of Descartes and Sir Isaac Newton. The best way to use this to your advantage is to simply be aware of what's happening. You can't exactly *force* yourself to cheer up when you're feeling sad, but you can acknowledge your feelings and look at what your body is doing. If you're feeling stressed at work, for instance, take a moment to think to yourself, *I am feeling stressed*. Then look at what your body is doing. How is your posture? Are you sitting down? Do you need to take a walk to make yourself feel better? Your emotions, both negative and positive, can be a trigger for your daily walking habit.

With these tools handy, you're well on your way to making daily walking automatic. Automating a healthy activity, creating space for it in your life, and finding ways to improve all increase the likelihood that you will remain consistent in your walking. Consistency results in positive health outcomes, which in turn reinforces new habits. In other words, you've started a healthy habit loop that isn't going away any time soon.

Consciously Sticking to Your Walking Routine

Starting a whole new routine is a daunting task, and it may not come naturally at first. While you're working on creating new small and unconscious habits to bolster your walking routine, there are also several other steps you can take to make your new routine easier to do. Before you work out, consider the following:

- **Adjusting your mindset**

Walking as an activity can be a little boring and repetitive, especially if you walk down the same trail at the same time of day for every exercise. But wait... doesn't consistency in time and location build sustainable habits? How can a person make walking interesting without ruining all of the efforts you put into building a habit? The answers to these questions depend on you, the resources you have, and your imagination. If you're into bird-watching, for instance, try incorporating that interest into your exercise—this isn't a workout, this is a bird-watching expedition! Listening to media like podcasts or audiobooks is another great example of this. It's important to keep in mind that walking and exercising are never a punishment, and your new habits can be made into something that's fun and enjoyable.

- **Anticipating how walking will make you feel**

Before you walk, try to remember a time when walking or exercising made you feel good. Did your energy and outlook improve after the strength training exercise you performed the other day? Did playing outside with your dog last week make you feel warm and fuzzy? Try to apply this feeling to the exercise you're about to do. Not only will this motivate you to go through with your workout, but it will also start to build positive associations in your mind.

- **Prioritizing your new routine**

Unconsciously turning your walking routine into a habit is great, but it also takes some concerted effort at first. If it's between sitting at your desk for lunch and walking to your nearest takeout restaurant, sticking to your guns means doing the latter. Ultimately, it's up to you, and you need to make space for your health in every way you can.

- **Walking with people you love**

Walking with a buddy (from pets to friends or family) is perhaps one of the best ways to keep yourself accountable. You don't have to walk with someone else every day, but scheduling a few walks with someone you love can do wonders for your motivation. Walking groups are also a great way to accomplish this, as well as meeting people with common interests in your area. Platforms like Meetup or Nextdoor are perfect for connecting with your local community, and getting some steps in while you're at it!

Another great way to jump-start your routine is to motivate yourself with positive reinforcements. If you do well and stick to your workout plan, reward yourself with something you like! As long as you don't go crazy with your rewards, small and consistent reinforcements will ultimately boost your motivation. In fact, these reinforcements can actually be integrated into your walk. For me, this looks like walking to my local bakery once a week and picking up some fresh bread—it never fails to get me excited, and having a tangible (and edible) reward at the end makes the process of walking even more encouraging! Another great motivator for walking can be adding fun, new additions to your routine. This can include new shoes, a pedometer, or even new headphones. Motivation can also take the form of games or bets with friends, which is a good option if you're more of a competitive person.

With all that being said, failure is unavoidable. Everyone falls off the wagon every so often, and we all have our flaws. You're human, after all! Circumstances change, and it isn't always your fault if you are not able to walk every day. When you miss a day, don't punish yourself. Guilt, contrary to popular belief, is not an effective motivator when it comes to health. One 2022 survey from Strava found that over 25% of American women under 35 name guilt as a primary reason why they exercise (McCarthy, 2022), and yet this doesn't seem to translate into long-term fitness changes. Another study found that nearly three-quarters of people who set fitness resolutions fall off the exercise wagon before they meet their goals (Ries, 2020), meaning that all those who exercise due to feeling guilty aren't getting anywhere.

It's also worth mentioning that chronic feelings of guilt or shame hanging over your head can make you feel terrible, worsening your mental health and making you even less motivated to get up and get moving. Believe me, I can speak from experience! Fitness instructor

Kelsey Wells agrees with this sentiment, telling one Australian media outlet that working out because of guilt or shame is, "'neither productive or healthy'" (McCarthy, 2022). In these situations, it's helpful to think of what you'd say if you were your own best friend. Chances are, you'd probably advise yourself to take it easy, and try again tomorrow. The entire point of exercising and building healthy habits is to make you feel better, and guilt-tripping yourself does not accomplish this.

I found that a lot of my motivation comes from walking with other people (or pets). Despite being a self-described independent and strongly disciplined introvert, the mental low points that occasionally roll around are hard to escape. During these periods, getting myself up and out the door becomes a huge mountain to climb. I suddenly have no sense of *why* walking would be good for me, and I just can't convince myself otherwise. For anyone who can relate to this sentiment, you also know that escaping negative emotional loops can be incredibly hard. This is perhaps why, at my lowest, my trusty German Shorthaired Pointer came to my rescue. Since integrating walking into my daily life, I've found that reaching out to family, friends, neighbors, and even coworkers is the best way to get myself off the couch. All it takes is a quick text message, and before I know it, I'm getting my shoes laced up because I know someone is going to be knocking at my door soon. Accountability can be a scary word sometimes, implying that you've done something wrong. However, in this instance, accountability can perhaps be replaced with *support*. The biggest source of support in our lives often comes from our networks of loved ones and acquaintances, dogs included.

The renowned philosopher Søren Kierkegaard once said, "Everyday, I walk myself into a state of well-being [and] walk away from every illness. I have walked myself into my best thoughts, and I know of no thought so burdensome that one cannot walk away from it" (GoodReads, n.d.-d). No matter how discouraged you're feeling, and no matter how low your motivation levels are, there's always room for exercise, if even just a handful of minutes. Learning how to improve your physical and mental health, break out of those negative mental loops, and reach your health goals begins with making the leap from stillness to movement.

CONCLUSION

At this point, you have all the knowledge you'll ever need to start a healthy and sustainable walking routine. Unlike other sports or fitness fads, you'll never need a playbook for walking, and you could even start right now! You've also learned about the dangers of a sedentary lifestyle, as well as the physical and mental benefits of walking for just a short period every day. These benefits include:

- lowering your blood pressure
- keeping off excess weight
- reducing your risk for certain kinds of cancer
- lowering your chances for developing osteoporosis

- helping you sleep better
- improving several cognitive functions like memory, emotional management, and creative and analogical thinking
- preventing type 2 diabetes
- protecting yourself from metabolic diseases, heart conditions, and injuries

These can all be achieved with a quick walk every day. You also know how to start choosing your optional gear, what to look for in walking shoes, and how to stay safe on the road. You know about the importance of your posture and the effects it can have on your body, and you are also aware of what to look for in a good walking setting. No matter where you decide to walk, be it an indoor art gallery or a beachside trail, you are well-equipped to handle whatever is thrown your way—and you also have the tools to motivate yourself and keep your routine sustainable. When you inevitably fall off the walking-workout wagon, dust yourself off and try again. Simply place one foot in front of the other, rinse, and repeat for amazing long-term health improvements!

If this book inspired your health journey in any way, I would encourage you to pass it on. Writing a good review can help the next person jump-start their journey to becoming a walking workout expert, as well as spreading good health and fitness knowledge to a wider audience. Building a happier and healthier world starts with building a happier and healthier you!

REFERENCES

AAPSM explains running shoe anatomy. (n.d.). American Academy of Podiatric Sports Medicine. https://www.aapsm.org/runshoe-running-anatomy.html

About heart disease. (2019). U.S. Centers for Disease Control and Prevention. https://www.cdc.gov/heartdisease/about.htm

Advanced Neurotherapy PC. (2020, June 19). *4 reasons why walking outside benefits the brain.* advancedneurotherapy.com. https://www.advancedneurotherapy.com/blog/2015/09/10/walking-outside-brain

Advantages and disadvantages of treadmill use for exercise and pain relief. (2021, August 25). Seattle Neuro & Spine Surgery. https://seattleneuro.com/advantages-and-disadvantages-of-treadmill-use-for-exercise-and-pain-relief

Ali, S. (2022, January 31). *A quarter of US adults are physically inactive: CDC report.* The Hill. https://thehill.com/changing-america/wellbeing/longevity/592061-a-quarter-of-us-adults-are-physically-inactive-cdc

America's walking: Pre-walk warm-up routine. (n.d.). Public Broadcasting System. https://www.pbs.org/americaswalking/health/healthprewalk.html

Ammenheuser, M. (2022, April 22). *10 surprising benefits of walking.* My Southern Health. https://www.mysouthernhealth.com/benefits-of-walking

Aschwanden, C. (2022, January 19). *When the last thing you want to do is exercise.* The New York Times. https://www.nytimes.com/2022/01/19/well/move/habits-motivation-exercise.html

At-home fitness test. (2021, January 14). SPOTEBI. https://www.spotebi.com/fitness-tips/at-home-fitness-test

Ayeh-Datey, R. (2022, September 2). *When did yoga originate?.* Live Science. https://www.livescience.com/when-did-yoga-originate

AZquotes. (n.d.). *Erin Gray quote.* azquotes.com. https://www.azquotes. com/quote/522934

Bberkley. (2022, April 27). *Fitness: A brief history.* The Social and Health Research Center. https://sahrc.org/2022/04/fitness-a-brief-history

Bergland, C. (2015, June 12). *Hippocrates was right: "Walking is the best medicine".* Psychology Today. https://www.psychologytoday.com/us/blog/the-athletes-way/201506/hippocrates-was-right-walking-is-the-best-medicine

Bolitho, C. (n.d.). *What to wear hiking.* REI. https://www.rei.com/learn/expert-advice/how-to-choose-hiking-clothes.html

Boogaard, K. (2021, December 26). *How to write SMART goals.* Work Life by Atlassian. https://www.atlassian.com/blog/productivity/how-to-write-smart-goals

Boyer, M. (2021, February 2). *How your posture is affecting your life.* Campus Recreation. https://campusrec.wfu.edu/2021/02/how-your-posture-is-affecting-your-life

BrainyQuote. (n.d.). *Lee Haney quotes.* brainyquote.com. https://www.brainyquote.com/quotes/lee_haney_295632

Bratman, G. N., Anderson, C. B., Berman, M. G., Cochran, B., de Vries, S., Flanders, J., Folke, C., Frumkin, H., Gross, J. J., Hartig, T., Kahn, P. H., Kuo, M., Lawler, J. J., Levin, P. S., Lindahl, T., Meyer-Lindenberg, A., Mitchell, R., Ouyang, Z., Roe, J., Scarlett, L., Smith, J. R., Van Den Bosch, M., Wheeler, B. W., White, M. P., Zheng, H., & Daily, G. C. (2019). Nature and mental health: An ecosystem service perspective. *Science Advances, 5*(7). https://doi.org/10.1126/sciadv.aax0903

Bratman, G. N., Hamilton, J. P., Hahn, K. S., Daily, G. C., & Gross, J. J. (2015). Nature experience reduces rumination and subgenual prefrontal cortex activation. *Proceedings of the National Academy of Sciences of the United States of America, 112*(28), 8567–8572. https://doi.org/10.1073/pnas.1510459112

Bremner, L. (2022, April 1). *Consistency – The missing link to achieving your health & fitness goals.* Luke Bremner Fitness. https://yourpersonaltraineredinburgh.com/power-of-consistency

Bumgardner, W. (2021, October 19). *10 walking mistakes to avoid.*

Verywell Fit. https://www.verywellfit.com/walking-mistakes-to-avoid-3435576

Bumgardner, W. (2022, August 3). *When it's time to get new walking shoes.* Verywell Fit. https://www.verywellfit.com/when-should-i-replace-my-walking-shoes-3436325

Bussel, M. (2018, June 12). *5 ways sitting is killing your nerves.* Neuropathic Therapy Center; Loma Linda University Health. https://lluh.org/services/neuropathic-therapy-center/blog/5-ways-sitting-killing-your-nerves

Butler, S. (n.d.). *The health benefits of hula hooping.* The Joint Chiropractic. https://www.thejoint.com/california/downey/downey-31109/243640-health-benefits-hula-hooping

Cafasso, J. (2017, June 2). *Understanding foot supination: Causes, treatment, and exercises.* Healthline. https://www.healthline.com/health/supination

Carlson, S. A., Adams, E. K., Yang, Z., & Fulton, J. E. (2018). Percentage of deaths associated with inadequate physical activity in the United States. *Preventing Chronic Disease, 15.* https://doi.org/10.5888/pcd18.170354

Chertoff, J. (2018, November 8). *What are the benefits of walking?.* Healthline. https://www.healthline.com/health/benefits-of-walking#lowers-blood-sugar

Choi, K. W., Chen, C.-Y., Stein, M. B., Klimentidis, Y. C., Wang, M.-J., Koenen, K. C., & Smoller, J. W. (2019). Assessment of bidirectional relationships between physical activity and depression among adults. *JAMA Psychiatry, 76*(4), 399–408. https://doi.org/10.1001/jamapsychiatry.2018.4175

Clear, J. (2015, February 24). *The 5 triggers that make new habits stick.* James Clear. https://jamesclear.com/habit-triggers

Cler, C. (2015, October 29). *Before mats were modern.* Wanderlust. https://wanderlust.com/journal/before-mats-were-modern

Compton, J. (2021, May 14). *3 people share how a walking routine helped them lose weight — and feel happier.* TODAY.com. https://www.today.com/health/how-establish-walking-routine-lose-weight-feel-happier-t218481

Conderino, S. E., Feldman, J. M., Spoer, B., Gourevitch, M. N., & Thorpe, L. E. (2021). Social and economic differences in neighborhood walkability across 500 U.S. cities. *American Journal of Preventive Medicine, 61*(3), 394–401. https://doi.org/10.1016/j.amepre.2021.03.014

Conway, I. (2010, April 20). *Stepping out the Afghan way*. The Irish Times. https://www.irishtimes.com/news/health/stepping-out-the-afghan-way-1.654699

Cook, S. D., Kester, M. A., & Brunet, M. E. (2016). Shock absorption characteristics of running shoes. *The American Journal of Sports Medicine, 13*(4), 248–253. https://doi.org/10.1177/036354658501300406

Cronkleton, E. (2019, December 17). *16 cooldown exercises you can do after any workout*. Healthline. https://www.healthline.com/health/exercise-fitness/cooldown-exercises#after-running

Curry, D. (2023, January 9). *Fitness app revenue and usage statistics (2023)*. Business of Apps. https://www.businessofapps.com/data/fitness-app-market

Dailey, T. (2022). *How to pick a good sock: Top 5 socks for athletes*. Freeland Foot & Ankle Clinic. https://www.freelandfoot.com/blog/top-five-podiatrist-recommended-socks-for-athletes.cfm

Dalleck, L. C., & Kravitz, L. (2019). The history of fitness. unm.edu. https://www.unm.edu/~lkravitz/Article%20folder/history.html

Dalli, K. (2022, August 16). *Consistency may be more important for workouts than duration of exercise, study finds*. ConsumerAffairs. https://www.consumeraffairs.com/news/consistency-may-be-more-important-for-workouts-than-duration-of-exercise-study-finds-081622.html

DeAngelis, T. (2022, November 1). *Want to boost your mental health? Take a walk*. American Psychological Association. https://www.apa.org/monitor/2022/11/defeating-depression-naturally

Different types of walking. (n.d.). Decathlon United Media. https://www.decathlon-united.media/media/sportfolios/different-types-of-walking.html

Disease/condition: Overpronation: What it is, causes & treatment. (n.d.).

Cleveland Clinic. https://my.clevelandclinic.org/health/diseases/22474-overpronation

Do most Americans still live where they grew up?. (n.d.). North American Moving Services. https://www.northamerican.com/infographics/where-they-grew-up

Doyle, A. (2022, September 7). *What is the average number of work hours per week?.* The Balance. https://www.thebalancemoney.com/what-is-the-average-hours-per-week-worked-in-the-us-2060631

Ducharme, J. (2019, February 28). *Spending just 20 minutes in a park makes you happier. Here's what else being outside can do for your health.* Time. https://time.com/5539942/green-space-health-wellness

The Editors of Prevention. (2017, October 25). *The amazing health benefits of walking outside every day.* Prevention. https://www.prevention.com/fitness/g20500099/benefits-of-walking-1

Eisenbraun, K. (2018, May 11). *6 benefits of walking outdoors every day.* Garcia Weight Loss. https://garciaweightloss.com/blog/6-benefits-walking-outdoors-every-day

Exercise: Starting a walking program. (n.d.). Berkeley; University Health Services. https://uhs.berkeley.edu/health-topics/exercise-starting-walking-program

Feder, S. (2019, November 8). *The fear of fat: Our last acceptable bias.* YES! Magazine. https://www.yesmagazine.org/social-justice/2019/11/08/fat-bias-fear-weight-stigma

5 reasons your workout should include a warm up & cool down. (2019, November 9). Paul H Broyhill Wellness Center. https://wellness.apprhs.org/5-reasons-your-workout-should-include-a-warm-up-cool-down

5 surprising benefits of walking. (2022, August 25). Harvard Health Publishing. https://www.health.harvard.edu/staying-healthy/5-surprising-benefits-of-walking

Flat feet health issues by advanced foot & ankle specialists. (2015, February 12). Advanced Foot and Ankle Specialists. https://www.advancedfootdocs.com/blog/2015/02/why-flat-feet-are-bad-for-your-health

Forcum, T., & Hyde, T. (2004, May 24). *Guidelines for buying walking shoes*. Spine-health. https://www.spine-health.com/wellness/exercise/guidelines-buying-walking-shoes

Garrick, N. (2017, April 7). *Osteoporosis*. U.S. National Institute of Arthritis and Musculoskeletal and Skin Diseases. https://www.niams.nih.gov/health-topics/osteoporosis

Gilpin, S. (n.d.). *The benefits of walking outside*. fdoa.org. https://www.fdoa.org/index.php?option=com_dailyplanetblog&view=entry&year=2021&month=09&day=08&id=20:the-benefits-of-walking-outside

GoodReads. (n.d. -a). *A quote by Confucius*. goodreads.com. https://www.goodreads.com/quotes/405004-roads-were-made-for-journeys-not-destinations

GoodReads. (n.d.-b). *A quote by Hippocrates*. goodreads.com. https://www.goodreads.com/quotes/9225741-if-you-are-in-a-bad-mood-go-for-a

GoodReads. (n.d.-c). *A quote by Shannon L. Alder*. goodreads.com. https://www.goodreads.com/quotes/736100-life-always-begins-with-one-step-outside-of-your-comfort

GoodReads. (n.d.-d). *A quote by Søren Kierkegaard*. goodreads.com. https://www.goodreads.com/quotes/336809-above-all-do-not-lose-your-desire-to-walk-everyday

Green facts. (n.d.). University of Michigan. https://hr.umich.edu/sites/default/files/green-facts-%202015.pdf

Green L. (2021, May 7). *10 ways to build an actually sustainable workout routine you love*. SELF. https://www.self.com/story/fitness-resistance-building-sustainable-workout-program

Gremaud, A. L., Carr, L. J., Simmering, J. E., Evans, N. J., Cremer, J. F., Segre, A. M., Polgreen, L. A., & Polgreen, P. M. (2018). Gamifying accelerometer use increases physical activity levels of sedentary office workers. *Journal of the American Heart Association, 7*(13). https://doi.org/10.1161/jaha.117.007735

Haq, A., Svobodová, J., Imran, S., Stanford, C., & Razzaque, M. S. (2016). Vitamin D deficiency: A single centre analysis of patients from 136 countries. *The Journal of Steroid Biochemistry and Molecular Biology, 164*, 209–213. https://doi.org/10.1016/j.jsbmb.2016.02.007

Hayes, S. (2004). *Am I too fat to be a princess? Examining the effects of popular children's media on preschoolers' body image*. STARS; University of Central Florida. https://stars.library.ucf.edu/cgi/view content.cgi?referer=&httpsredir=1&article=4747&context=etd

HealthPartners. (2022, June 3). Health risks of a sedentary lifestyle and how to make changes. HealthPartners Blog. https://www.healthpartners.com/blog/health-risks-of-sedentary-lifestyle/

Health risks | Obesity Prevention Source. (2012). Harvard T.H. Chan. https://www.hsph.harvard.edu/obesity-prevention-source/obesity-consequences/health-effects

Health risks of an inactive lifestyle. (n.d.). U.S. National Library of Medicine. https://medlineplus.gov/healthrisksofaninactivelifestyle.html

HealthyWomen. (2011, December 4). *6 tips for indoor walking*. healthywomen.org. https://www.healthywomen.org/content/article/6-tips-indoor-walking

Hip flexors. (n.d.). Physiopedia. https://www.physiopedia.com/Hip_Flexors

Hoonan, R. (2021, January 27). What's the best way to cool down after exercise?. Right as Rain by UW Medicine. https://rightasrain.uwmedicine.org/body/exercise/how-to-cool-down

Hori, H., Ikenouchi-Sugita, A., Yoshimura, R., & Nakamura, J. (2016). Does subjective sleep quality improve by a walking intervention? A real-world study in a Japanese workplace. *BMJ Open, 6*(10). https://doi.org/10.1136/bmjopen-2016-011055

How to walk with proper form and technique for fitness. (n.d.). maine.gov. https://www.maine.gov/mdot/challengeme/topics/docs/2019/may/How-to-Walk-with-Proper-Form-and-Technique-for-Fitness.pdf

How walking can boost your mental health. (2022, May 5). Health Assured. https://www.healthassured.org/blog/how-walking-can-boost-your-mental-health

It's easy being green: Walking vs. driving is a no-brainer. (2008, July 2). The Center for American Progress. https://www.americanprogress.org/article/its-easy-being-green-walking-vs-driving-is-a-no-brainer

Jain, S. (n.d.). *12 surprising signs that you are not moving enough*. Naturally Yours. https://naturallyyours.in/blogs/blog/12-surprising-signs-that-you-are-not-moving-enough

Jaret, P. (2021, September 17). *High blood pressure*. WebMD. https://www.webmd.com/hypertension-high-blood-pressure/guide/high-blood-pressure

Karunaharamoorthy, A. (2022, July 19). *Tensor fasciae latae muscle*. Kenhub. https://www.kenhub.com/en/library/anatomy/tensor-fasciae-latae-muscle

Klein, B. (2021, June 24). *Types of walking styles explained*. CityScene Magazine. https://www.cityscenecolumbus.com/arts-and-entertainment/types-of-walking

Kuzma, C. (2020, July 22). *14 ways to make your daily walk feel more like a walking workout*. SELF. https://www.self.com/story/walking-workout-tips

Laskowski, E. R. (2021, September 22). *How much should the average adult exercise every day?*. Mayo Clinic. https://www.mayoclinic.org/healthy-lifestyle/fitness/expert-answers/exercise/faq-20057916

Ledochowski, L., Ruedl, G., Taylor, A. H., & Kopp, M. (2015). Acute effects of brisk walking on sugary snack cravings in overweight people, affect and responses to a manipulated stress situation and to a sugary snack cue: A crossover study. *PLOS ONE, 10*(3), e0119278. https://DOI.org/10.1371/journal.pone.0119278

Lefave, S. (2020, March 26). *Yes, it's okay to take a walk outside during coronavirus*. Oprah Daily. https://www.oprahmag.com/life/health/a31944589/benefits-of-walking

Lisa, A. (2023, January 6). *The biggest diet and exercise fads of the past century*. Cheapism. https://blog.cheapism.com/fitness-fads

LOliva. (2022, July 19). *Mental health benefits of walking outside in nature*. Cano Health. https://canohealth.com/news/blog/mental-health-benefits-of-walking-outside

LVMC Staff. (2021, April 30). *Importance of good posture*. Lompoc Valley Medical Center. https://lompocvmc.com/blog/124-healthy-living/1763-importance-of-good-posture

Maguire, L. G. (2019, August 1). *Analogical thinking: A way to produce

REFERENCES | 183

creative ideas. Medium. https://medium.com/the-creative-mind/analogical-thinking-a-way-to-produce-creative-ideas-510cb9923fd0

Mansour, S. (2021a, January 21). *Headed out for a walk? Warm up with these 9 stretches.* TODAY.com. https://www.today.com/health/9-exercises-warm-you-walk-or-run-cold-t206295

Mansour, S. (2021b, November 9). *3 meditative walks that will boost your mood and shift your mindset.* TODAY.com. https://www.today.com/health/3-walking-meditations-will-boost-your-mood-t238229

Massey, J. (2015, June 1). *Mind-body medicine its history & evolution.* Naturopathic Doctor News & Review. https://ndnr.com/mindbody/mind-body-medicine-its-history-evolution

Mayo Clinic Staff. (2021a, May 11). *Get walking with this 12-week walking schedule.* Mayo Clinic. https://www.mayoclinic.org/healthy-lifestyle/fitness/in-depth/walking/art-20050972

Mayo Clinic Staff. (2021b, May 19). *Walking: Trim your waistline, improve your health.* Mayo Clinic. https://www.mayoclinic.org/healthy-lifestyle/fitness/in-depth/walking/art-20046261

Mayo Clinic Staff. (2022a, January 27). *Walking: Make it count with activity trackers.* Mayo Clinic. https://www.mayoclinic.org/healthy-lifestyle/fitness/in-depth/walking/art-20047880

Mayo Clinic Staff. (2022b, November 3). *HDL cholesterol: How to boost your 'good' cholesterol.* Mayo Clinic. https://www.mayoclinic.org/diseases-conditions/high-blood-cholesterol/in-depth/hdl-cholesterol/art-20046388

McCallum, K. (2021, October 19). *Is lactic acid buildup really what causes muscle soreness after a workout?.* Houston Methodist. https://www.houstonmethodist.org/blog/articles/2021/oct/is-lactic-acid-buildup-really-what-causes-muscle-soreness-after-a-workout

McCarthy, A. (2022, June 30). *One easy way to overcome exercise guilt when you skip a workout.* The Latch. https://thelatch.com.au/exercise-guilt/

Mendez Colmenares, A., Voss, M. W., Fanning, J., Salerno, E. A., Gothe, N. P., Thomas, M. L., McAuley, E., Kramer, A. F., & Burzynska, A. Z. (2021). White matter plasticity in healthy older adults: The effects of aerobic exercise. *NeuroImage, 239,* 118305. https://doi.org/10.1016/j.neuroimage.2021.118305

Metabolic syndrome - Symptoms and causes. (2021, May 6). Mayo Clinic. https://www.mayoclinic.org/diseases-conditions/metabolic-syndrome/symptoms-causes/syc-20351916

Meyer, A. (2022, June 14). *5 outdoor walking workouts.* Verywell Fit. https://www.verywellfit.com/outdoor-walking-workouts-how-tos-and-tips-5324672

Miller, J. C., & Krizan, Z. (2016). Walking facilitates positive affect (even when expecting the opposite). *Emotion, 16*(5), 775–785. https://doi.org/10.1037/a0040270

Mooney, C. (2015, June 29). *New research suggests nature walks are good for your brain.* Washington Post. https://www.washingtonpost.com/news/energy-environment/wp/2015/06/29/fixating-or-brooding-on-things-take-a-walk-in-the-woods-for-real

Most polluted cities | State of the air. (2021). American Lung Association. https://www.lung.org/research/sota/city-rankings/most-polluted-cities

Move your body. (n.d.). Cancer Council Australia. https://www.cancer.org.au/cancer-information/causes-and-prevention/diet-and-exercise/move-your-body

Mukhwana, J. (2021, November 25). *Types of walking styles and how to use them for maximum health benefits.* BetterMe Blog. https://betterme.world/articles/types-of-walking-styles

Munsell, S. (2018, March 6). *Common walking problems: Part 1 of 6 from overstriding to gliding.* Dynamic Vitality. https://dynamicvitality.com/1199-2

Nazario, B. (2021, April 22). *Fitness and exercise: Surprising signs you're not moving enough.* OnHealth. https://www.onhealth.com/content/1/exercise_surprising_signs_not_moving_enough

Obesity. (2020, February 21). World Health Organization. https://www.who.int/health-topics/obesity#tab=tab_1

Oppezzo, M., & Schwartz, D. L. (2014). Give your ideas some legs: The positive effect of walking on creative thinking. *Journal of Experimental Psychology: Learning, Memory, and Cognition, 40*(4),

1142–1152. https://doi.org/10.1037/a0036577

Park, J. H., Moon, J. H., Kim, H. J., Kong, M. H., & Oh, Y. H. (2020). Sedentary lifestyle: Overview of updated evidence of potential health risks. *Korean Journal of Family Medicine, 41*(6), 365–373. https://doi.org/10.4082/kjfm.20.0165

Physical inactivity a leading cause of disease and disability, warns WHO. (2002, April 4). World Health Organization. https://www.who.int/news/item/04-04-2002-physical-inactivity-a-leading-cause-of-disease-and-disability-warns-who

Plantar fasciitis - Symptoms and causes. Mayo Clinic. (2022, January 20). Mayo Clinic. https://www.mayoclinic.org/diseases-conditions/plantar-fasciitis/symptoms-causes/syc-20354846

Quinn, E. (2020, February 19). *Test your upper body fitness with the push-up test.* Verywell Fit. https://www.verywellfit.com/push-up-test-for-upper-body-strength-and-endurance-3120272

Quinn, E. (2022, August 29). *VO2 max testing: How the test is done and what the results mean.* Verywell Fit. https://www.verywellfit.com/what-is-vo2-max-3120097

Rabbitt, M., Phoenix, K., & Haase, M. (2022, October 27). *12 major benefits of walking, according to experts.* Prevention. https://www.prevention.com/fitness/a20485587/benefits-from-walking-every-day

Ralph Waldo Emerson quotes III. (n.d.). NotableQuotes. http://www.notable-quotes.com/e/emerson_ralph_waldo_iii.html

Raman, R. (2018, April 28). *How to safely get vitamin D from sunlight.* Healthline. https://www.healthline.com/nutrition/vitamin-d-from-sun

Ries, J. (2020, January 3). *Trying a new workout in the new year? Why you shouldn't go full throttle.* Healthline. https://www.healthline.com/health-news/you-probably-shouldnt-go-full-throttle-at-the-gym

Ritchie, D. (2021, June 17). *Sedentary lifestyle: 10 signs you aren't active enough.* Calendar. https://www.calendar.com/blog/sedentary-lifestyle-10-signs-you-arent-active-enough

"A river cuts through rock, not because of its power, but because of its persistence." (n.d.). The Foundation for a Better Life. https://www.passiton.com/inspirational-quotes/7524-a-river-cuts-through-rock-not-because-of-its

Rogers, K., & Young, B. (2017, October 10). *Using pedometers as a motivational tool to increase physical activity. Be Broncho Fit!* https://blogs.uco.edu/wellnesscoachingprogram/2017/10/10/using-pedometers-as-a-motivational-tool-to-increase-physical-activity

Rogers, M. (2021, August 24). *The importance of being consistent with exercise.* National Federation of Professional Trainers. https://www.nfpt.com/blog/consistent-in-exercise

Roland, A. (n.d.). *Try online yoga classes for senior adults.* Wellness360 Magazine. https://wellness360magazine.com/try-online-yoga-classes-for-senior-adults

Roland, J. (2020, January 16). *How to walk properly with good posture.* Healthline. https://www.healthline.com/health/how-to-walk

Romero, S. (2022, February 14). *Pedestrian deaths spike in U.S. as reckless driving surges.* The New York Times. https://www.nytimes.com/2022/02/14/us/pedestrian-deaths-pandemic.html

Safety tips for exercising outdoors for older adults. (n.d.). U.S. National Institute on Aging. https://www.nia.nih.gov/health/exercising-outdoors

Saint-Maurice, P. F., Graubard, B. I., Troiano, R. P., Berrigan, D., Galuska, D. A., Fulton, J. E., & Matthews, C. E. (2022). Estimated number of deaths prevented through increased physical activity among US adults. *JAMA Internal Medicine, 182*(3), 349–352. https://doi.org/10.1001/jamainternmed.2021.7755

Sanders, J. L. (2010, June 11). *Understanding the impact of shoe insoles and midsoles.* Podiatry Today. https://www.hmpgloballearningnetwork.com/site/podiatry/blogged/understanding-impact-shoe-insoles-and-midsoles

Schmidt, S. (2023, January 25). *What are the different types of walking workouts?.* wisegeek. https://www.wisegeek.net/what-are-the-different-types-of-walking-workouts.htm

Schmitt, A. (2017, September 27). *Public health experts give America an "F" on walkability.* Streetsblog USA. https://usa.streetsblog.org/2017/09/27/public-health-experts-give-america-an-f-on-walkability

Schultz, A. (2018, December 13). *Are treadmill workouts really as effective as running outside?*. GQ. https://www.gq.com/story/treadmill-runs-vs-outside-runs-explained

Serotonin: What is it, function & levels. (n.d.). Cleveland Clinic. https://my.clevelandclinic.org/health/articles/22572-serotonin

7 tips to motivate yourself to exercise. (n.d.). Long Island Spine Specialists. https://www.lispine.com/blog/7-tips-to-motivate-yourself-to-exercise

Siddiqui, S. V., Chatterjee, U., Devvarta, K., Siddiqui, A., & Goyal., N. (2008). Neuropsychology of prefrontal cortex. *Indian Journal of Psychiatry, 50*(3), 202–208. https://doi.org/10.4103/0019-5545.43634

Stanners, M. (2021, September 20). *Benefits of walking: Reasons why walking is so good for your mental health*. Step One. https://www.steponecharity.co.uk/benefits-walking-mental-health

Steinhilber, B. (2018, May 4). *Why walking is the most underrated form of exercise*. NBC News. https://www.nbcnews.com/better/health/why-walking-most-underrated-form-exercise-ncna797271

Tamkins, T. (2019, January 16). *19 moving stories from people who used exercise to change their life*. BuzzFeed News. https://www.buzzfeednews.com/article/theresatamkins/how-exercise-can-save-your-life

Teale, C. (2020, October 15). *US cities less walkable than international counterparts: study*. Smart Cities Dive. https://www.smartcitiesdive.com/news/us-cities-less-walkable-than-international-counterparts-study/587046

10 walking mistakes – Are you walking wrong?. (n.d.). Camelback Sports Therapy. https://camelbacksportstherapy.com/10-walking-mistakes-are-you-walking-wrong

3 surprising risks of poor posture. (2021, February 15). Harvard Health Publishing. https://www.health.harvard.edu/staying-healthy/3-surprising-risks-of-poor-posture

12 benefits of walking. (n.d.). Arthritis Foundation. https://www.arthritis.org/health-wellness/healthy-living/physical-activity/walking/12-benefits-of-walking

Type 2 diabetes - Symptoms and causes. (2022, November 19). Mayo

Clinic. https://www.mayoclinic.org/diseases-conditions/type-2-diabetes/symptoms-causes/syc-20351193

U.S. and world population clock. (2022). United States Census Bureau. https://www.census.gov/popclock

"A walk in nature, walks the soul back home." —Mary Davis. (n.d.). The Foundation for a Better Life. https://www.passiton.com/inspirational-quotes/8107-a-walk-in-nature-walks-the-soul-back-home

Walking and breathing with rhythm. (n.d.). Vancouver Island Health Authority. https://www.islandhealth.ca/sites/default/files/2018-05/copd-walking-breathing.pdf

Walking and mental health. (n.d.). The Mindshift Foundation. https://mindshift.org.au/walking-and-mental-health

Walking for good health. (2012). Better Health Channel. https://www.betterhealth.vic.gov.au/health/healthyliving/walking-for-good-health

Walking gets the feet moving, the blood moving, the mind moving. - Terri Guillemets. (2020, November 27). andiquote.org. https://andiquote.org/quote/8644/

Wang, F., & Boros, S. (2020). The effect of daily walking exercise on sleep quality in healthy young adults. *Sport Sciences for Health, 17,* 393–401. https://doi.org/10.1007/s11332-020-00702-x

Weir, K. (2020, April 1). *Nurtured by nature.* American Psychological Association. https://www.apa.org/monitor/2020/04/nurtured-nature

Wetzler, T. (2021, July 15). *Health & fitness apps continue to trend upwards in 2021.* Adjust. https://www.adjust.com/blog/health-fitness-apps-trend-upwards-in-2021

What makes a neighborhood walkable. (n.d.). Walk Score. https://www.walkscore.com/walkable-neighborhoods.shtml

White matter disease: What it is, symptoms & treatment. (n.d.). Cleveland Clinic. https://my.clevelandclinic.org/health/diseases/23018-white-matter-disease

Why warming up and cooling down is important. (2016, December 15). Tri-City Medical Center. https://www.tricitymed.org/2016/12/warming-cooling-important

Zare, H., Gaskin, D. D., & Thorpe, R. J. (2021). Income inequality and obesity among US adults 1999–2016: Does Sex Matter?. *International Journal of Environmental Research and Public Health*, *18*(13), 7079. https://doi.org/10.3390/ijerph18137079

Printed in Great Britain
by Amazon